Bodies in Transition in the Health Humanities

In recent years, the transitioning body has become the subject of increasing scholarly, medical, and political interest. This interdisciplinary collection seeks to enable productive dialogue about bodily transformation and its many potential meanings and possibilities.

Recent high-profile sex transitions, such as Bruce Jenner's transformation into Caitlyn, have contributed to a proliferation of public and private debates about the boundaries of personal identity and the politics of gender. Sexual transition is only one possible type of bodily transformation, and bodies that change forms vex many binaries that underpin daily life such as male/female, gay/straight, well/unhealthy, able/disabled, beautiful/ugly, or adult/child. When transformations and transitions involve trauma, illness, injury, surgery, or death, bodies can become culturally and socially illegible and enter the realm of abjection or even horror. Health humanities, a recent revision of medical humanities that includes patients and other nonphysicians, provides an interdisciplinary lens through which to read such bodily transformation and its representation in public culture. The authors of the essays in the present volume situate their work in this interdisciplinary space to enable productive dialogue about bodily transformation and its meanings in artistic, literary, visual, and health discourses. The chapters discuss non-normative bodies from eighteenth-century France to present-day Iran and investigate narratives of cancer, aging, anorexia, AIDS, intersexuality, transsexuality, viruses, bacteria, and vaccinations.

This collection will be of key interest to faculty and students in women's studies/ gender studies, cultural studies, studies of visual and material culture, medical/health humanities, disability studies, and rhetorics of science, health, and medicine, and will be a useful resource for scholars across interdisciplinary fields of study.

Lisa M. DeTora is Associate Professor of Writing Studies and Rhetoric and Director of STEM Writing at Hofstra University. She has published widely on scientific and medical affairs and the medical humanities. In addition, she is the editor of *Heroes of Film, Comics, and American Culture* (2009) and *Regulatory Writing: An Overview* (2017).

Stephanie M. Hilger is Professor of Comparative Literature and German at the University of Illinois at Urbana-Champaign. She is the author of *Women Write Back* (2009) and *Gender and Genre* (2014). She is also the (co-)editor of *New Directions in Literature and Medicine Studies* (2017) and *The Early History of Embodied Cognition* (2015).

Bodies in Transition in the Health Humanities

Representations of Corporeality

Edited by
Lisa M. DeTora and Stephanie M. Hilger

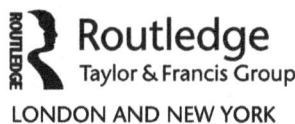

Routledge
Taylor & Francis Group

LONDON AND NEW YORK

First published 2020
by Routledge
2 Park Square, Milton Park, Abingdon, Oxon OX14 4RN

and by Routledge
605 Third Avenue, New York, NY 10017

First issued in paperback 2021

Routledge is an imprint of the Taylor & Francis Group, an informa business

British Library Cataloguing in Publication Data
A catalogue record for this book is available from the British Library

Library of Congress Cataloging-in-Publication Data
Names: DeTora, Lisa, 1966- editor. | Hilger, Stephanie M. (Stephanie Mathilde), editor.
Title: Bodies in transition in the health humanities : representations of corporeality / edited by Lisa M. DeTora and Stephanie M. Hilger.
Description: London ; New York : Routledge, 2019. | Includes bibliographical references and index.
Identifiers: LCCN 2019009500 (print) | LCCN 2019010602 (ebook) | ISBN 9781351128742 (master) | ISBN 9780815356066 (hardback : alk. paper)
Subjects: | MESH: Human Body | Attitude | Disease | Infection | Gender Identity
Classification: LCC RA776.5 (ebook) | LCC RA776.5 (print) | NLM HM 636 | DDC; 613–dc23
LC record available at https://lccn.loc.gov/2019009500

ISBN 13: 978-1-03-209140-2 (pbk)
ISBN 13: 978-0-8153-5606-6 (hbk)

Typeset in Sabon
by Taylor & Francis Books

Contents

Figures

Contributors

Lisa M. DeTora is Associate Professor of Writing Studies and Rhetoric and Director of STEM Writing at Hofstra University. She also serves as guest faculty in medical humanities for the Hofstra Northwell Medical School. Her research focuses on biomedicine, trauma, young adult literature, and embodiment. She has published dozens of articles in scientific and medical affairs, as well as medical humanities. She is the editor of *Heroes of Film, Comics, and American Culture: Essays on Real and Fictional Defenders of Home* (2009), the co-editor of the Graphic Narrative Research Committee proceedings of the 2016 International Comparative Literature Association meeting, and the editor of *Regulatory Writing: An Overview* (2017).

Katelyn Dykstra holds a Ph.D. from the Department of English, Theatre, Film and Media at the University of Manitoba, Canada, where she is an instructor in the Women's and Gender Studies Program. Her dissertation engages contemporary representations of intersex in film and literature. She has forthcoming publications in two collaborative projects: on the value of gender-play workshops for trans youth (with Dr. Fenton Litwiller) and on *Game of Thrones* and feminism (with Karalyn Dokurno). She is also a book reviewer for the *Winnipeg Free Press* and is involved in community building initiatives in southeast Manitoba.

Carl Fisher is currently Senior Director, Academic Personnel at the California State University Office of the Chancellor, after serving as Professor of Comparative Literature and Chair of the Department of Human Development at California State University, Long Beach. His specialization is eighteenth-century studies, and he has published on Rabelais, Rousseau, Defoe, Fielding, Sterne, Chekhov, and graphic satire in the eighteenth century. He is working on two scholarly projects in Health Humanities, one on nineteenth-century women writing about medicine, and another on the representation of illness in graphic novels.

Rebecca Garden is Associate Professor of Bioethics and Humanities at SUNY Upstate Medical University in Syracuse, NY. She has published widely in journals such as *New Literary History, Disability Studies Quarterly*, the

Journal of General Internal Medicine, and the *Journal of Clinical Ethics*, as well as in the *Journal of Medical Humanities* and *Literature and Medicine*. She is Executive Director of the Consortium for Culture and Medicine, an inter-institutional collaboration in Syracuse.

Barbara Grüning is Assistant Professor of Sociology at the University of Milan, Bicocca. She was a post-doc research fellow at the University of Bologna (2009–2018) and at the University of Lüneburg (2009). She was a visiting scholar at the ZDF in Potsdam (2007), the Technische Universität of Berlin (2014 and 2016), and the "Zentrum Marc Bloch" in Berlin (2017). Her research interests include the sociology of knowledge, the sociology of memory, space studies, body studies, and narrative studies.

Stephanie M. Hilger is Professor of Comparative Literature and German at the University of Illinois at Urbana-Champaign. Her research focuses on eighteenth-century British, French, and German literature and culture; she is currently working on a book project entitled "Liminal Bodies: Hermaphrodites in the Eighteenth Century." She is the author of *Women Write Back: Strategies of Response and the Dynamics of European Literary Culture, 1790–1805* (2009) and *Gender and Genre: German Women Write the French Revolution* (2014). She is also the editor of *New Directions in Literature and Medicine Studies* (2017) and co-editor of *The Early History of Embodied Cognition from 1740 to 1920* (2015).

Jens Lohfert Jørgensen (b. 1968) is Associate Professor in Scandinavian Literature at Aalborg University, Denmark. He is the author of the monograph *Signs of Disease* (2013), which reads the works of the Danish author Jens Peter Jacobsen as a signifying process corresponding to the progression of tuberculosis. He has also published articles in Danish and international journals on bacteriology and modernism and on the field of literature and medicine. He has edited an issue of the journal *Academic Quarter* on medical humanities and is the investigator and former leader of the research network *Nordic Network for Studies in Narrativity and Medicine*.

Elizabeth Lanphier is a Ph.D. Candidate in Philosophy at Vanderbilt University, where she also trains with the Clinical Ethics Consult Service at the Center for Biomedical Ethics and Society. Lanphier earned a master's degree in Narrative Medicine from Columbia University. Previously Elizabeth worked for Doctors Without Borders/Médecins Sans Frontières and the International Center for AIDS Care and Treatment Programs in their headquarters offices while also providing field support to programs in francophone Africa. She recently contributed a chapter on humanitarian aid in conflict settings to the *Cambridge Handbook on Just War* entitled "Humanitarianism: Neutrality, Impartiality, and Humanity" (2018).

Yianna Liatsos is Lecturer in English at the University of Limerick, Ireland. She has published essays on critical theory and post-apartheid literature and her current research focuses on embodiment and narrative identity. She is working on the topic of empathic imagination and narrative medicine and is completing a monograph on the discourse of choice in relation to motherhood.

Adnan Mahmutović is a Bosnian-Swedish writer and literary scholar in the fields of postcolonial studies, comics studies, world literature, creative writing, and also eco criticism. His works include *The Craft of Editing* (2018), *Visions of the Future in Comics* (2016), *Ways of Being Free* (2012), *How to Fare Well and Stay Fair* (2012), and *Thinner than a Hair* (2010).

Jennifer A. Malkowski explores the rhetoric of health and medicine. She has engaged a variety of public issues geared at preserving agency and restoring collective action through improved policy communication. She has partnered with health care professionals and organizations to improve policy communication in response to health risks. Her work has appeared in *Health Communication* and the *Journal of Medical Humanities* and is forthcoming in the *Rhetoric of Health and Medicine*.

Peter Martin is University Professor of Human Development and Family Studies at Iowa State University. He received a Ph.D. in Human Development and Family Studies from The Pennsylvania State University and a Doctor of Philosophy in Psychology from the University of Bonn, Germany. His research is concerned with adult development and aging. Dr. Martin has published articles on personality, psychological well-being, and successful aging. He is a Fellow of the Gerontological Society of America and the current Editor-in-Chief of the *Journal of Adult Development*.

Najmeh Moradiyan-Rizi is a doctoral candidate in the Department of Film and Media Studies at the University of Kansas. She holds a Graduate Certificate from KU's Department of Women, Gender, and Sexuality Studies, an M.A. in Film and Media Study from SUNY Buffalo, and B.F.A. and M.A. degrees in Cinema from Tehran University of Art. She is the author of "Iranian Women, Iranian Cinema: Negotiating with Ideology and Tradition" (in the *Journal of Religion and Film*, 2015) and "The Acoustic Screen: The Dynamics of the Female Look and Voice in Abbas Kiarostami's *Shirin*" (in *Synoptique*, 2016).

Denise Ask Nunes holds an M.A. in English Literature from Stockholm University. Her research focuses on the question of the animal and on ecocritical literature. Research from her master's thesis, "Maxime Mirandra in Minimis: Reimagining Swarm Consciousness and Planetary Responsibility," has been published in *ImageText* and *Visions of the Future in Comics*.

Nora Martin Peterson is Associate Professor of French at the University of Nebraska, Lincoln. She received a Ph.D. in Comparative Literature from Brown University. Her book, *Involuntary Confessions of the Flesh in Early Modern France* appeared in 2016 as part of the "Early Modern Exchanges" series with the University of Delaware Press. Her research interests include the body and medicine in early modern literature and culture, Marguerite de Navarre's *Heptaméron*, early modern women's writing, embodiment, travel narratives, fairy tales, comparative literature, and literary theory.

Angelika Vybiral is a lecturer in German language and Austrian culture and history in the Department of German Studies at the Comenius University in Bratislava, Slovakia, and teaches French literature and Media Studies in the Department of Romance Studies at the University of Vienna, Austria. She currently holds a doctoral fellowship from the Austrian Academy of Sciences. Her articles on gender and medicine have appeared in *Astheure, Edinburgh German Yearbook, Trajectoire, Vom Geheimen und Verborgenen: Enthüllen und Entdecken in der Medizin*, and *Wissen—Ordnung—Geschlecht*.

Acknowledgements

Bodies and medical/health humanities have been at the center of our individual research agendas for some years. We have published on a broad range of historical periods and contexts, ranging from eighteenth-century German plays to present-day American graphic novels and comics. While we are scholars of literature and rhetoric, our work bridges the humanities and the sciences in the form of health humanities and bioethics.

The initial idea for this specific collection on intelligible states of corporeality emerged from several seminars we (co-)organized at the American Comparative Literature Association (ACLA) annual meetings, some of which were co-sponsored by the Graphic Narrative Research Group of the International Comparative Literature Association (ICLA). Other influences and scholarly communities that informed this volume include the Northeast Modern Language Association, Columbia University's Program in Narrative Medicine, and the Rhetoric Society of America (RSA). In various seminars and workshops, we met and engaged scholars at all career stages, from different corners of the world. Each of us was, in some way wrestling with the meaning of bodies that did not quite fit normative ideals. The productive exchange in each seminar and in our broader research networks highlighted the necessity for this type of volume. The goal of this collection was to integrate ideas about the transitioning body, based on our realization that the many different permutations of "transition" are often inextricably linked with the central issue of gender binaries.

Such a project as this would not have been possible without the support of both of our institutions, Hofstra University and the University of Illinois at Urbana-Champaign, which supported our travels to the above-mentioned conferences and provided logistical support for our work on the volume.

We would like to thank the authors for their inspiring contributions and the editors at Routledge for their support and guidance throughout the publication process.

Last but not least, we would like to acknowledge the formative influences of scholars and friends like Marcelline Block of Princeton University and Baruch College, whose earlier volume *Gender Scripts in Literature and Medicine* first brought some of the contributors to the current volume together in print. Anne

Hudson Jones' presence at the first seminar we organized was crucial for our development as medical/health humanities scholars. Carl Fisher of the California State University has been a steady mentor and friend to the ACLA medical humanities community for over a decade. In Lisa's case, formative influences also include the meninge community of physicians, scientists, and scholars among whom she worked for over a decade, as her earlier publications attest. Stephanie is thankful to the Medical Humanities community at Illinois, which provided her with an intellectually stimulating framework for her own transition from a literary to a health humanities scholar.

Foreword

In a way that may be true for many health humanities scholars, my life is shaped by embodied transformation and my work derives from a compelling need for an intellectual framework for that experience of transition. My journey to my position as a health humanities scholar and educator and dedicated champion of this growing field begins with a story of illness and its impact on a tightly knit family of friends. As a scholar who has made narrative central to her research and education, a story is not surprisingly central to my entrance into the discipline.

It was my birthday and my friends Robert and Douglas took me to Coney Island to celebrate. We rode the Cyclone. For me, it was the first time on any roller coaster, and it was breathtaking and delirious, whirling and whipping me around above the midway, the sea, and our beloved sprawling city.

When the ride was over, and I was clambering out of my seat, I heard a voice over the PA system repeating my name. Bewildered, I looked up and saw the ride attendant and everyone on the ride staring at me. Then the attendant began to croon the birthday song into the microphone. My friend Robert was smiling demurely as he sang. He had arranged that for me.

After much laughter (them) and blushing wildly (me), we rode the Cyclone again, screaming and laughing as we careened. On the way home, Robert grew silent and then lay down in the back seat of the car. I thought he was queasy from the rides. We soon realized he was seriously ill. He developed severe fever and was hospitalized. Then I learned that Robert was dying. He was HIV positive and experiencing the symptoms of his first—and worst—opportunistic infection, cryptococcal meningitis, a dangerous disease.

It was the early 1990s and there was not yet any life-saving treatment for AIDS. Robert had known of his diagnosis for almost a year but had deliberately kept it from me until I had completed my master's degree in literature and been accepted into Columbia's English PhD program—a place where I had persisted despite the punishing forty percent attrition rate.

Robert survived his bout with cryptococcal meningitis but with serious damage to his health. He soon developed dementia associated with AIDS. As Robert grew sicker, my research interests shifted from early twentieth-century literature, with a focus on African American history and culture, to literature that involved illness, death, and trauma. My historical frame shifted gradually back through time to the eighteenth century, when there was very little medicine could do biologically and the treatment of illness was instead primarily social and cultural.

For me and Robert's other friends, his disease, the complications, and the processes of dying were not medical matters but a shared experience of illness. We also were suffering and needed healing, and healing would not come through medicine, but through the sense we could make of the trauma AIDS generated. From my perspective, Robert was not infected with cryptococcal meningitis; he was suffering from brain fever. He did not develop AIDS-related dementia; he was slowly going mad, and so was I. His illnesses and transformations bewildered me. The medical explanations of the overworked physicians at St. Vincent's Hospital never dispelled the dread and disorientation that began to haunt my days. Instead, I found solace and eventually a means of making meaning of Robert's transformations in literature that made suffering and disease fundamental to individual identity and community formation. I explored literature where the boundaries of metaphor broke down, so that literature itself became a treatment, a form of inoculation. By inflicting suffering in a mediated form, literature might enable the reader to survive the epidemic.

Robert died, and I survived his loss by developing a practice of making meaning—and re-making my world—through my engagement with literature and culture. I discovered and coopted for my own use literary genres such as the conversion narrative—which pivoted upon the breakdown of the self through illness and novels that made disease and treatment the foundation of individual and social development. These literary treatments helped me to reconstruct and redefine Robert's dissolution and my own mourning within a revised historical and cultural framework.

Soon, I discovered a field that encompassed what had felt like an isolated enterprise. After my friend's death and while working on my dissertation, I saw a job posting sent to English department graduate students by Rita Charon, Director of Columbia medical school's Program in Narrative Medicine, an internal medicine physician who earned her PhD in literature (from Columbia) later in her career. I was hired as Program Coordinator and Managing Editor of the journal, *Literature and Medicine* (I eventually became Associate Director of the program). My first duties included working with author Michael Ondaatje during his year as writer-in-residence at the medical school, a position ideally suited to him given his profound literary engagements with loss, trauma, and embodied suffering in novels like *The English Patient* and *Anil's Ghost*. I coordinated his readings and seminars, as well as the reading series he organized with cultural stars like Joan Didion, Paul Auster, Art Spiegelman, and Walter Murch. Ondaatje's seminars and the talks and readings he organized brought these authors into conversation with clinicians—nurses, social workers, and other health professionals, as well as physicians—and medical students. I was immersed in seminar discussions of texts that worked through trauma and mourning more than disease and medicine itself. In seminars funded by the National Endowment for the Humanities, I explored the mechanisms of these texts and theorizations of the discipline in the company of founding members of

Narrative Medicine, such as the literary and film scholar Maura Spiegel, philosopher Craig Irvine, clinician and scholar Sayantani Dasgupta, and psychiatrist Eric Marcus, as well as Rita Charon.

Charon established a lecture series called Narrative Medicine Rounds, establishing literary studies and writing as an aspect of medical school culture positioned to be on a par with the "grand rounds" lectures in all of the established departments, which residents, students, hospital staff, and faculty attend. She hosted talks with medical humanities experts such as Allan Peterkin, MD, psychiatrist at University of Toronto, and his colleague Guy Allen, PhD, professor of writing at University of Toronto with a background in expressive writing. Peterkin and Allen co-led a writing group for people affected by HIV/AIDS that was a hybrid form of a writer's workshop and group therapy sessions. I began to perceive the vast range of possibilities of a cross-disciplinary field that addresses not only medicine but also that which has been medicalized and which medicine cannot heal.

Rita Charon is one of the founders of the field of medical humanities, a person who, like humanities scholars such as Joanne Trautmann Banks, Anne Hudson Jones, Kathryn Montgomery, Ann Hunsaker Hawkins, and Suzanne Poirier, saw the relevance of the study of literature and creative writing to the theories and practices of medicine (Charon et al., "Literature and Medicine"). Charon's Program in Narrative Medicine evolved from her success at creating within Columbia's College of Physicians and Surgeons a culture that welcomed her experimentation with literary studies and writing. Charon had already instituted the Parallel Chart project (Charon 155–174; Klein) which gave medical students the opportunity to write about and discuss their experiences of patients, to explore all the things that did not fit into the notes they were taught to write in the tightly scripted patient chart (which are today constrained even further thanks to the electronic health record system, which has replaced handwritten notes on a paper chart with a series of clicks on drop-down menus). Having won over her school's curriculum committee, Charon instituted this project for all first-year students. Collaborating with a wide range of faculty and staff as group facilitators, Charon earned the support of key institutional stakeholders for the ideas and practices of what she calls Narrative Medicine. This approach asserts, in part, that the ability to analyze and investigate the details of a poem or story—such as William Carlos Williams' "Use of Force" (part of the medical humanities canon)—correlates with the ability to recognize, interpret, and respond to subtle symptoms or social cues—such as hierarchies of expertise or signs of abuse—in order to identify and respond empathically to suffering in patients. In recognition of the currency of medical education and its emphasis on core "competencies" (e.g., "Patient Care," "Medical Knowledge," and "Professionalism"), Charon insists on the need for "narrative competency" in medical education and practice, a canny strategy for making humanities-based knowledge and skill fundamental to medical practice.

Through my experiences working in a medical school—including reading over a hundred interviews conducted by a medical anthropologist with medical students in their first year "on the wards," involving innumerable stories of the students witnessing and also experiencing suffering, harm, and loss in clinical care—I came to comprehend the role the humanities might play as a critical supplement to healthcare pedagogy and practice. I saw how discussing a text could create a space for reflecting on clinical encounters in a way that was not possible in the clinical setting itself, whether during the patient–provider encounter (with its severe restrictions on time), or even in a staff session devoted to reviewing challenging issues in the clinic. Discussing a text rather than an actual problem or "case" provides a protective layer of distance from the immediacy of charged or controversial issues in the clinic and even diminishes somewhat the relatively strict hierarchy of roles and thus representation of perspectives. Talking about a clinical issue or case often involves assigning responsibility for error or parsing differences of opinion along with the weight of roles and authority. Talking about a literary text allows participants to voice opinions and perspectives with a greater claim to equality of expertise and to address topics that are often controversial in the clinic but more freely discussed when somewhat abstracted from the realm of immediate responsibility.

When I became more involved with literature seminars for medical students, I saw the value of engaging them in a practice that deepened their interpretive skills and their ability to deal with ambiguities and nuances and to interpret language in social as well as interpersonal contexts, helping them to process the experiences on the ward that generated their haunting stories and to find words for the encounters that they could not initially describe. One of the founders of the medical humanities, Joanne Trautmann Banks, defended the value of literary study as relevant to "scientific truth" by observing that fiction "necessarily deals in shades of truth: in ambiguities and nuances" (Trautmann Banks 33). For Trautmann Banks (the first literary scholar to hold an appointment in a medical school), the medical humanities helps students to develop critical reading practices, and in doing so, expands their capacity to make meaning of the suffering they witness and experience. To her, reading fiction takes clinicians beyond mere *"illustrations* of the medical subject" and exposes them to *"illuminations"* (35) that develop their "tolerance for ambiguity, for coming to conclusions where the data are incomplete or capable of being interpreted variously" (36). Trautmann Banks understands that:

> [T]o teach a student to read, in the fullest sense, is to help train him or her medically. To ask the medical student what is being said here … [to] look at words in their personal and social contexts and when several things are being said at once—is to prepare him or her for the doctor–patient encounter.
>
> (36)

Health humanities scholars and their students in healthcare continue to demonstrate the importance of these cross-disciplinary practices (Charon et al., "Close Reading").

The more I understood the culture of medicine, the more I appreciated how the Narrative Medicine seminars encouraged exploration of social and interpersonal issues in medicine. Still, I continued to be skeptical of the lack of representation in the seminars of those who experience illness, disability, and difference in the context of healthcare, those defined and medicalized as *patients*. While we often had a wide range of medical roles and professions represented in our discussion, including administrative staff, we rarely had people who identified (much less who rejected identification) as patients participating in the conversation. Perhaps the text was to stand in for the experience of patients. I had not yet read Anne Hudson Jones's critique and complication of the way medical humanities scholars' deployment of interpretive skills might coalesce physician authority by reducing patients to a text subject to their interpretation and mastery (Jones). I often felt like the sole representative of patients' perspectives, not because I identified as an ill or disabled person or someone who had a more than infrequent experience with healthcare, but rather because I was a "civilian," left out of the specialized language and references to medical cultures and consistently struck by the strangeness of medicine's practices, norms, and values. I was clearly an outsider and marked as less knowledgeable and credible in a world that had sharply defined borders, despite my privileged status as a graduate student in an Ivy League school. I was thus able to witness the ways that, despite the leveling nature of a book group meeting or seminar discussing a literary text, hierarchy and claims to authority and expertise persisted.

Rita Charon's success in creating a medical school culture that embraced Narrative Medicine also meant that the power structures inherent in the culture of medicine were reinforced in certain ways *by* the culture of Narrative Medicine, despite the fact that the focus on texts written by and representing non-physicians was inherently a leveling approach. By the time I became involved in the program, the seminars Charon organized were eagerly attended by deans and department and division chairs and some of the leading specialists in fields such as neurology and cardiology, as well as promising medical students, and wise and seasoned (although less celebrated) nurses and social workers. A writer covering Ondaatje's residency for the *New Yorker*'s "Talk of the Town" column attended the seminars where clinicians recognized as leaders in their field engaged in fine-grained discussions of texts such as William Maxell's *So Long, See You Tomorrow*, Penelope Fitzgerald's *The Blue Flower*, and Anne Carson's *Glass, Irony, and God*. The excitement and impact created by such a successful programming of literary seminars at a medical school created some countercurrents to the goal of the project, which was to deepen understandings of people's experiences of loss, illness, and disability.

Sometimes we navigated these countercurrents in the seminars. When discussing passages of Carson's poetry, in which the narrator describes the impact of her father's dementia on her interactions with him, I saw some resonances with my own experience with my friend Robert, and I made an observation to the group about the ways Carson's poetry represents intact fragments of the former self that remain like capsules of that identity that open up for a momentary re-connection before disappearing again into confusion, forgetfulness, or simply profound alterity: "Flaps down! I cry," the narrator says to her father, who was a World War II airman. "His black grin flares once and goes out like a match" (Carson 27). The renowned neurologist quickly dismissed my perception as a misunderstanding of stray neurological activity rather than a momentary resurgence of identity. The light may flicker on, he said, but I can assure you that nobody's home. One of his colleagues affirmed his observation, and the conversation moved on. The neurologist was unaware of how personally invested I was in my observation and probably would have been more careful in his response if he had known. I probably should have reclaimed the thread of the discussion instead of silently stewing in the wake of what felt like a curt dismissal. Nonetheless, it demonstrated to me that the ability to analyze and have a robust discussion about literature does not necessarily entail empathy (a foundational assumption of medical humanities as a humanistic or at least humanizing enterprise), nor does it necessarily raise questions about the hierarchy of expertise in health and healthcare, which is to me the point of studying literature produced by and representing the perspectives of non-physicians.

Part of the maturation of the field of health humanities—and, for some, its development beyond *medical* humanities—has been an insistence on challenging the norms and hierarchies of medicine and healthcare. Most contemporary health humanities scholars—including those working in social science discourses and disciplines—are not constricted to the narrow focus on the interpersonal interactions of the clinic, but rather are engaging in broader social, political, and historical analyses. This kind of critical approach to medicine and to the field of medical humanities itself are part of the history of the field. Such an approach is less well known to a non-specialist audience, in which literature is primarily understood as a means of improving the patient–provider relationship, ostensibly by developing empathy for patients, and as a means for "self-care" for providers (for example, as respite from the "real" work of patient care). Without a critique of the medicalization of illness and disability and an analysis that encompasses social forces, this approach reinforces the structures of medical authority, rather than analyzing them and establishing more equitable frameworks for power and expertise. Health humanities scholarship—such as the work found in this volume—is increasingly focused on the social, political, and historical dimensions of health, illness, disability, and healthcare, the inequalities in society as well as in interpersonal interactions in the clinic, and the ways in which those inequalities are embodied, biologized, and/or materialized.

Making questions of power and privilege central to health humanities inquiry is complicated for those of us working from academic positions within the institutions of medicine and healthcare. We sometimes make our colleagues uncomfortable when we challenge the structures and instrumentalities that enable hierarchies of power and expertise. Attempts to allay that discomfort may undermine the potentially radical methodologies and practices of the humanities. Since being hired as a professor of bioethics and humanities at a health sciences university, I have found that the critiques of medicine and public health that I had adopted through my graduate school education in English did not prepare me to contend with the usually well-intentioned clinicians, educators, and bioethicists who participated in a system that was nonetheless set up to more or less exploit the patient's narrative for the benefit of the system and its participants— patients themselves and their intimate circles and caregivers.

I saw (and still see) issues that to me are best characterized by Foucauldian understandings of the clinical gaze, biopower, and biopolitics, or orientalism, or, in a more focused critique of health humanities itself, by anthropologist Michael Taussig's suspicion of "humanistic reform-mongering" that enables more precise disciplinary control of patients (Taussig). These critical frameworks haunt me in productive ways, and I continuously work against the way that humanities are instrumentalized as a "fast track to patients' perspectives on illness and healthcare" (as some in my own institution have described Narrative Medicine) and something like literary case studies that *illustrate* rather than *illuminate* ethical or clinical issues in healthcare. Because my institution has not yet recognized and accepted the importance of the health humanities, the relevance of studying literature must be defended by virtue of its ability to perform as if it were a bioethics case or a clinical case scenario or at least provide specific background information in the way that a journal article might.

The critical and ethical goals of the health humanities are further complicated for those who go up for tenure and promotion in healthcare institutions where decisions about health humanities scholars are typically made by clinicians and basic scientists, who may be confused by the lack of grant funding and who look at numbers of publications (medical research generates more short articles than the humanities) and "impact factors" rather than the length and depth of essays, and who do not consider books to have the same level of rigor and significance as peer-reviewed articles. There are expectations of health humanities scholars publishing in clinical and bioethics journals, which may involve decisions by reviewers who are unfamiliar with and sometimes suspicious of critiques of medical authority. (During the extensive revise and resubmit process that I endured with one clinical medical journal, the editor deleted every single use of the word *power*—four times in all—until I painstakingly negotiated for two instances to remain). Many health humanities scholars in medical and health science institutions are asked to provide assessments of and evidence for the value of the health humanities. Those of us who are members of the Health Humanities Consortium and its listserv share examples of assessments, but also arguments against reducing the benefits of our research and pedagogy to what can be empirically measured, a debate with which most in the humanities are increasingly familiar. Health humanities scholars and educators who are located in medical, nursing, and health professions schools experience innumerable explicit and subtle pressures to fit in with the norms and expectations of a culture that does not always welcome critique, where foundational arguments about marginalized embodiments need to be made again and again and are often met with skepticism and resistance, so that moving forward with more complex and nuanced analyses is repeatedly deferred.

Given these challenges and barriers, health humanities scholars in healthcare institutions—and, more importantly, those affected by medicine and public health and its influences—benefit enormously from the contributions of scholars in humanities and social science departments, such as the authors in this collection. These scholars complicate understandings of expertise and cross boundaries among disciplines, discourses, and genres; among bodies, minds, other forms of materiality, and discourses; and among science and other modes of knowledge and culture, opening up new ways of knowing the body and its relationship to others and to the world. They reveal the historical and social dimensions of what medicine and science represent as empirical. This form of health humanities shapes medicine—including medical practice and education—through analyses of issues that have long been medicalized but are being reclaimed by those whose bodies and cultures are at stake. In many ways, this form of health humanities circumvents or supplements medicine, performing what I describe elsewhere as "critical healing" through critical theoretical and activist approaches to health, public health, diagnosis, disability, and embodiment (Garden). Scholars and activists working outside of medicine and public health may be in a better position to keep those who are most subject to its influence in the center of research and practice. They also provide resources and can hold accountable those of us working on the institutional "inside" of medicine; for example, my involvement with the field of disability studies provides a significant counterweight to the forces of "humanistic reform-mongering" in medicine. Nonetheless, as health humanities baccalaureate programs grow in popularity—offering certificates, concentrations, majors, and minors—scholars working in those institutions will need to navigate something like "humanistic program-mongering" designed to attract as well as "reform" pre-health students. This reality argues for developing connections with health humanities scholars (as well as students and practitioners) in medicine and public health.

I encourage health humanities scholars and practitioners to more fully understand that medicine can be both a "medical industrial complex" and a complex culture, to recognize the ways in which distinctions between "patients" and "providers" and perceived hierarchies break down upon closer examination (e.g., many students and practitioners have first-hand or otherwise intimate relationships to illness and disability), and to forge alliances with those who can share knowledge, expertise, and strategies that might contribute to transformations beyond merely reforms (whether that be with people who seek and are subject to healthcare, practitioners, or the scholars on the fringes). The emphasis on disciplinary as well as embodied transitions, such as this volume makes evident, reveals and redefines diverse forms of embodiment, health, and healing.

There are many ways that those involved with the theories and practice of healthcare are simultaneously developing counternarratives and counterstructures that can begin to heal the social and embodied experiences of illness and injury, such as the trauma of medicalized difference and other forms of stigma. Decades after my friend Robert's death, I work with two activists who care for people dying of AIDS in their home and bring them into the classroom to teach my students about radical empathy and grassroots responses to disease and stigmatization. The courses that I teach weave the study of narrative and literature—with an emphasis on counternarratives, history, policy, and politics—together with an understanding that healing must involve the agency of those most affected. Robert's story—the story that I tell about him—remains central to my own practice of health humanities.

Works Cited

Carson, Anne. *Glass, Irony and God*. New York: New Directions, 2005.

Charon, Rita. *Narrative Medicine: Honoring the Stories of Illness*. Oxford: Oxford UP, 2006.

Charon, Rita, Nellie Hermann, and Michael J. Devlin. "Close Reading and Creative Writing in Clinical Education: Teaching Attention, Representation, and Affiliation." *Academic Medicine: Journal of the Association of American Medical Colleges* 91. 3 (2016): 345–350.

Charon, Rita, Joanne Trautmann Banks, Julia E. Connelly, Anne Hunsaker Hawkins, Kathryn Montgomery Hunter, Anne Hudson Jones, Martha Montello, and Suzanne Poirier. "Literature and Medicine: Contributions to Clinical Practice." *Annals of Internal Medicine* 122. 8(1995): 599–606.

Garden, Rebecca. "Critical Healing: Queering Diagnosis and Public Health through the Health Humanities." *Journal of Medical Humanities* (2018): 1–5.

Jones, Anne Hudson. "Reading Patients—Cautions and Concerns." *Literature and Medicine* 13. 2(1994): 190–200.

Klein, Joan. "Narrative Oncology: Medicine's Untold Stories." *Oncology Times* 25. 4(2003): 10–13.

Peterkin, Allan D. and Julie Hann. *Still Here: A Post-Cocktail AIDS Anthology*. Toronto: Life Rattle Press, 2008.

Taussig, Michael. "Reification and the Consciousness of the Patient." *The Nervous System*. New York: Routledge, 1992. 83–110.

Trautmann Banks, Joanne. "The Wonders of Literature in Medical Education." *MOBIUS: A Journal for Continuing Education Professionals in the Health Sciences* 2. 3(1982): 23–31.

1 Introduction

Bodies and Transitions in the Health Humanities

Lisa M. DeTora and Stephanie M. Hilger

During the United States bicentennial year, 1976, Bruce Jenner won the decathlon, reclaiming national athletic superiority at a significant juncture of Cold War politics: the Montreal Olympic Games, one of the few sites in which democratic and communist forms of government could claim victories. These sites of victory took place over bodies, the bodies of athletes as they transitioned to fame, broke world records, or succumbed to defeat. Jenner, later accorded the honor of adorning the Wheaties box in 1978, won his decathlon at a critical time, in the midst of a Space Race in which the U.S.A. was regularly outpaced by the Soviet Union. His intensive training program transformed his body from amateur to professional athlete and marked the first time a U.S. athlete trained to the level of state-sponsored Soviet counterparts (Carothers). Nearly forty years later, in 2015, Jenner marked another groundbreaking transition, from a transgendered man into a woman, Caitlyn—the first Olympic gold medalist to undertake such a transition (Brockes). Jenner's transitioning body has contributed to the proliferation of debates about the boundaries of personal identity and the politics of gender in popular culture and in scholarship.

Theoretical Approaches to Questions of Embodiment

One of the most essential questions underpinning lived experience is the implicit need to conform to gendered social expectations. In fact, gender binaries inform an understanding not only of personal lived experiences, but also of how we express those experiences in visual and cultural artifacts; thus, questions about the relationship of certain types of bodies and consequent identity occur in many registers. While highly politicized statements, such as the suggestion that gender is immutably fixed at birth (Green et al.), inform current public debates, more subtle questions also warrant close examination.

Recent psychological studies, such as the ones by Lauren Spinner and Laura Zimmermann, have found that children's toys send important messages about gender:

> Looking at how children play with toys that fall into gender stereotypes gives us a window on children's developing sense of what goes along with

being a boy or a girl. But it can also be an important indicator of what skills young children are acquiring as they play, and of whether their academic and professional horizons are comparatively wide—or whether they are already starting to rule things out for themselves.

(Klass n.p.)

In their studies, children's ideas about the fixity of gender norms were found to depend not merely on what toys they preferred, but also on how these choices were presented. In other words, children were less likely to see apparent gender identity and toy preferences as natural if they were offered different kinds of social messages. Significantly, the reporter who covered the story, Perri Klass, is a pediatrician whose reflective work situates her at an important intersection of humanistic and scientific understanding of embodied experiences. Although Klass' coverage suggests that these recent studies were scientific breakthroughs, they in fact build on a large body of existing knowledge.

Studies of the human body as a necessarily gendered entity entered scholarly, medical, and political discourse in the late twentieth century. Much of this attention grew out of feminist scholarship in the seventies and attendant studies of the epistemological significance of gender and its relationship to embodiment and corporeality. In the following decades, scholarly interest in the question of embodiment grew as can be seen in Anne Fausto-Sterling's *Myths of Gender: Biological Theories about Women and Men* (1985), Elaine Scarry's *The Body in Pain: The Making and Unmaking of the World* (1985), Judith Butler's *Bodies that Matter: On the Discursive Limits of Sex* (1993), Elisabeth Grosz' *Volatile Bodies: Toward a Corporeal Feminism* (1994), and Katie Conboy, Nadia Medina, and Sarah Stanbury's anthology, *Writing on the Body: Female Embodiment and Feminist Theory* (1997). These groundbreaking studies questioned a Western medical tradition that normalized the young man's body as a site of reference and thereby paved the way for the current understanding of gender in general and sexual transition in particular.

While sexual transition has become a crucial site for scholarly attention, it is only one possible type of bodily transformation. Debates about transgender persons' access to restroom facilities, for example, also foster discussions about broader questions concerning the human body and its place in society, such as issues of citizenship, morality, and the ethics of inclusivity and diversity. Bodies that change forms vex many binaries that underpin a common understanding of quotidian life: male/female, gay/straight, well/unhealthy, able/disabled, beautiful/ugly, and adult/child.

Butler's *Bodies that Matter*, in particular, posits a nuanced understanding of corporeal transformations and transitions that involve trauma, illness, injury, surgery, or death, in the context of gender as a fundamentally flawed binary. For Butler, trauma and illness can render bodily experiences both culturally and socially unrepresentable, unspeakable, thereby entering the realm of abjection or even horror. Butler comments on "abject, unliveable" bodies (3) that haunt the edges of representation, defying attempts to render their experiences into language. If we, like Butler, accept a Foucauldian construction of knowledge, one that assumes that knowledge only exists once it can be rendered into language, then a major challenge of current studies of the body is to account for the realm of abjection and the possibility for making such experiences meaningful.

The scholars who contributed to this volume examine debates on the body in different cultural, national, religious, and historical contexts and do so from a variety of perspectives: women's and gender studies, cultural studies, visual and material culture, health humanities, disability studies, and the rhetorics of science, health, and medicine. While subjective experiences of trauma and illness may appear to be of primarily personal significance, limited to the realm of psychological adjustment, the necessity for representing sickness, disability, and difference informs social interactions and the realm of medical practice.

Health Humanities

Medical humanities, a field of study that emerged in the 1970s and emphasized the moral dimension of medicine by seeking to bridge disciplinary divides, provides an interpretive lens through which to read representations of physical transformations due to trauma, illness, injury, surgery, or death. Scholars and teachers of medical humanities explore a wide range of interrelated topics: narrative medicine (the analysis of the narrative dimension of patients' and doctors' stories), the therapeutic uses of reading and writing literature (biblio- and scriptotherapy), writing about disease (pathography), the pedagogical uses of literature courses in the medical curriculum, the role of doctor-writers, the representation of the medical encounter in literary texts, the medical case history as a literary genre, changing literary depictions of disease, and the history of medicine, just to name a few of the most prevalent areas of inquiry. K. Danner Clouser, who was the very first full-time medical humanities faculty member, identified the goals of medical humanities as follows: that medicine draw on the humanities while the humanities examine the practices of medicine. In recent years, the term "health humanities" has gradually replaced "medical humanities" to address the reality that medicine affects more people than just physicians (Jones et al.). This semantic shift highlights the fact of multiple stakeholders in healthcare settings, including nonphysician healthcare professionals, patients, and relatives. In the past decade, as noted by Luca Chiapperino and Giovanni Boniolo, the pace of scientific discovery and technologically-informed practices has far outstripped that of considered philosophical, moral, and ethical approaches to biomedicine. A humanities-based intervention has therefore become more necessary than ever to recover the human in the practice of medicine and reflect on its treatments of bodies, especially those that vex received understandings of corporeality. The present collection expands on the work of existing volumes on health and medical humanities such as Ronald Carson and colleagues' *Practicing the Medical Humanities: Engaging Physicians and Patients* (2003), Thomas Cole and colleagues' *Medical Humanities: An Introduction* (2015), and Therese Jones and colleagues' *Health Humanities Reader* (2014). Unlike these more general collections, however, the authors in the present volume study one particular question: How the body is rendered representable or unrepresentable in various cultural contexts. We hope this volume will be a valuable resource in undergraduate and graduate curricula as well as for scholars across various interdisciplinary fields of study.

By casting health humanities as a site for critical thinking about bodily transformation and its representation in public culture, we can create room for the possibility raised by Gillie Bolton that mutual pressure might strengthen both medicine and the humanities. This type of inquiry necessarily leverages interdisciplinary practices, bridging not only biomedical sciences and the arts, but also varied theoretical and disciplinary approaches within the arts and letters. Thus, interdisciplinary approaches such as disability studies, cultural studies, or the history and rhetorics of science and biomedicine also underpin this growing discourse, allowing for an interrogation of the very terms that make certain bodies meaningful within the context of transition. The authors of the chapters in the present volume situate their work in this interdisciplinary space to enable productive dialogue about bodily transformation and its meanings within a context of scholarship that can accommodate various ways of making the body meaningful. Central to this discussion is the notion that bodily states and transformations cannot enter into the realm of knowledge unless they are rendered intellectually or socially intelligible at the margins of artistic, literary, visual, and health discourses.

In her foreword to the volume, Rebecca Garden describes her path to the health humanities by reflecting on the embodied experience of illness from the patient's perspective. She argues for the role that the humanities can play as a critical supplement to healthcare pedagogy and practice. Recuperating patients' perspectives through narrative medicine challenges the norms and hierarchies of medicine and healthcare. Garden's reflections frame the ethical issues raised by the chapters in this volume, which are grouped under three headings, each of which addresses a specific form of embodiment: modes of charting or mapping the body as a gendered entity, means of protecting the body from infection or invasion, and ways we document the body in the transition between life and death.

Charting Bodily Norms in Official and Educational Discourses

The first section, "Medical Models, Charts, and Institutional Narratives," considers medical and legal modes of describing people and bodies, particularly those that defy gender expectations, in official or public documents. The authors in this section examine the development of biomedical case studies and charting as well as ongoing critiques of those official discourses. Ultimately, these authors assert that the close examination and mapping of bodies that defied gender expectations formed the basis for our current understanding of gendered norms.

Angelika Vybiral examines the exhibition of female wax models in the historical-anatomical collection of the Viennese Josephinum, the Austrian medical academy, founded in 1784. Because early anatomical wax models were primarily male, the rarity of female forms in this medium makes them particularly significant for understanding debates regarding gender norms in the eighteenth century and beyond. Yet these norms hinged not so much on the existence of unequivocal gender binaries as on descriptions of bodies that called such binaries into question.

Gender norms and the eighteenth-century medical discourse on gender also stand at the center of Stephanie Hilger's essay on medical case studies about Michel-Anne Drouart, a so-called hermaphrodite. Drouart's case, like that of other sexually ambiguous people who served as medical models, appeared in court documents as well as the news media of the day. In the context of the Enlightenment's empirical endeavor to elucidate all mysteries of the natural world, scientists carefully examined, measured, and recorded all the details of Drouart's sexually ambiguous body. Yet this body, like that of other persons of ambiguous gender, thwarted scientific efforts to elucidate its workings. The failure to establish firm gender binaries contributed to a profound sense of epistemological anxiety that emerged from profound shifts in eighteenth-century structures of knowledge.

The medicalization of sexually ambiguous bodies continues today, as discussed in Katelyn Dykstra's essay on present-day intersex life narratives, published in the 2015 issue of the journal *Narrative Inquiry in Bioethics*. For Dykstra, these narratives resist medical discourse as represented by and established in the medical chart as an accepted and official documentation genre. Access to the medical chart permits persons whose gender does not neatly fit into binary categories to reclaim agency and form an activist community around the collective memorializing of their medical trauma.

The trauma caused by the medical treatment of non-normative bodies is also the focus of Najmeh Moradiyan Rizi's reading of *Be Like Others* (2008), a documentary on transsexuality in Iran. The author challenges the film's reductive approach to this issue, which aligns it with homosexuality, and highlights instead the complexities and particularities of sex change in the country. By questioning neo-Orientalist discourses, this essay foregrounds the complexity of the formation of transsexual identity in post-Revolutionary Iran, where gender, sexual, and cultural norms are constantly being negotiated and contested.

The connection between activism, gender expectations, and medical trauma is not limited to sexual transition or gender ambiguity. Resistance to the trauma caused by medical intervention is also the topic of Barbara Grüning's chapter on Italian anorexia sufferers' autobiographical narratives, which question the institutionalized spaces of centers for eating disorders and hospitals. The chapter explores the social and cultural environments of southern and northern Italian cities, the influence of Italian Catholic culture on gender roles, the authors' social status, and the historical context as central agents that shape both the women's spatial experience of their body and the ways this experience is narrated.

Infection, Invasion, and Protection

Section two, "Invasive Influences and Corporeal Integrity," considers representations of the body as a site of illness, infection, and transition in medical discourses, specifically in microbiology. While the primary transition of interest in these essays is between illness and health, representations of the body as a site of bacterial invasion or microbiological activities provide a second unifying theme.

The desire to reclaim control over a non-normative body informs Lisa DeTora's discussion of what she terms "the meningococcal body." Typical stories of meningococcal disease highlight disability, especially disfiguration among young women, and focus on vaccination as a preventative measure. DeTora juxtaposes this public health discourse with the narratives of Paralympian Amy Purdy, who describes her own transition through invasive meningococcal infection as a site of personal agency, and with medical narratives describing a normal meningococcal infection as not causing disease. In layering these stories, DeTora sees the existence of a certain type of "meningococcal body," one in which both material corporeality and gender identity are superpositioned and radically reframed outside of typical discourses of disability and vaccination.

Jennifer Malkowski examines vaccination as a newly gendered discourse following the introduction of the Human Papillomavirus (HPV) vaccine. While HPV affects both men and women, public health discourse gendered it as a female disease, equating it with cervical cancer, only one of the possible outcomes, as a result of limitations in the research used to support marketing. As a result of the sexualized casting of cervical cancer in popular culture, the reach and efficacy of the vaccine, which was approved by the FDA in 2006, has been severely limited. Yet more significantly, the HPV vaccine introduced a language of appropriate femininity into what had previously been a gender-neutral public health discourse.

The current focus on viruses has its antecedent in nineteenth- and early twentieth-century fears regarding the potentially destructive effects of bacteria, as Jens Lohfert Jørgensen shows in his contribution on modernist literature. At the same time that the new science of bacteriology contributed to a bacillophobia through hygienic campaigns, it also questioned the anthropocentric worldview by showing that humans exist in symbiosis with a seething multitude of non-human organisms.

A post-anthropocentric approach also shapes Adnan Mahmutović and Denise Ask Nunes' reading of filmmaker Ridley Scott's prequels to the original Alien tetralogy, *Prometheus* (2012) and *Alien Covenant* (2017). These prequels' quest for origins is tied to genetic manipulation and insemination. At the center stands the human, robot, alien trinity whose bodies come to intertwine and metamorphose, blurring boundaries between bodies, science, and divinity, thereby embodying a post-human worldview.

Death as Transition

The question of what it means to be human informs the essays in the third section of this volume, "Aging, Decline, and Death," which examines autobiographical documents by people enmeshed in the transition from life to death. Nora Martin Peterson and Peter Martin examine the writings of six-teenth-century French philosopher Michel de Montaigne on various moments of embodied transitions: a near-death experience, aging, cognitive decline, and loss. Successful aging, for Montaigne, is the acceptance of the transition from mind to body. And, Montaigne further argues, the relationship between the mind and body can be symbiotic, even during the process of dying.

The symbiosis between mind and body is also documented in the American artist Hannah Wilke's series of photographic self-portraits that she took during her treatment for terminal lymphoma in the 1990s. Elizabeth Lanphier considers Wilke's photographic self-portraiture as an illness narrative that situates the artist and the viewer in an ethical relationship of mutual meaning-making. Lanphier suggests that photographs and self-portraits, especially in the era of "selfie" culture, may be apt tools for supporting a responsive, creative, and intersubjective ethics of care for twenty-first century medicine.

The intersubjective dimension of establishing meaning in the face of illness is also explored in Yianna Liatsos' analysis of two memoirs written by a husband and wife on his diagnosis of terminal glioblastoma multiforme: Tom Lubbock's *Until Further Notice I am Alive* (2012) and Marion Coutts' *Iceberg* (2014). Liatsos examines the relational dimension of terminal disease and its doc-umentation, underlining the importance of health humanities in the recovery of the multitude of voices in a healthcare setting.

Finally, in the afterword to the volume, Carl Fisher reflects on the sig-nificance of the health humanities in the context of the expanding field of healthcare. Health humanities emphasizes attention to multidisciplinary view-points, including the study of psychological and sociocultural perspectives, and strives to develop skills of observation, analysis, empathy, and self-reflection, which are all crucial to encourage better healthcare practices. Fisher also traces his own journey in the health humanities in research and teaching. He outlines his pedagogical approach, which stresses that the arts provide the reader/viewer both opportunity for identification and distance in considering essential elements of the human experience.

Works Cited

Bolton, Gillie. "Boundaries of Humanities: Writing Medical Humanities." *Arts and Humanities in Higher Education* 7. 2(2007): 131–148.

Brockes, Emma. "Caitlyn Jenner on Transitioning: 'It Was Hard Giving Old Bruce Up. He Still Lives Inside Me'." *The Guardian*8 May 2017. www.theguardian.com/tv-and-radio/2017/may/08/caitlyn-jenner-bruce-transitioning-kardashians-reality-tv-star.

Butler, Judith. *Bodies That Matter: On the Discursive Limits of Sex*. New York: Taylor and Francis, 1993.

Carothers, Cassie. "1978 Flashback: Bruce Jenner, Wheaties, and the 'Breakfast of Cham-pions'." *Yahoo Food* 23 April 2015. www.yahoo.com/lifestyle/1978-flashback-bruce-jenner-wheaties-and-the-117171767386.html.

Carson, Ronald A., Chester R. Burns, and Thomas R. Cole, eds. *Practicing the Medical Humanities: Engaging Physicians and Patients.* Hagerstown: University Publishing Group, 2003.

Chiapperino, Luca and Giovanni Boniolo. "Rethinking Medical Humanities." *Journal of Medical Humanities* 35(2014): 377–387.

Cole, Thomas R., Nathan S. Carlin, and Ronald A. Carson. *Medical Humanities: An Introduction.* New York: Cambridge UP, 2015.

Conboy, Katie, Nadia Medina, and Sarah Stanbury. *Writing on the Body: Female Embodiment and Feminist Theory.* New York: Columbia UP, 1997.

Fausto-Sterling, Anne. *Myths of Gender: Biological Theories about Women and Men.* New York: Basic Books, 1985.

Green, Erica L., Katie Benner, and Robert Pear. "'Transgender' Could Be Defined Out of Existence Under Trump Administration." *New York Times* 21 October 2018. www.nytimes.com/2018/10/21/us/politics/transgender-trump-administration-sex-definition.html.

Grosz, Elizabeth. *Volatile Bodies: Toward a Corporeal Feminism.* Bloomington: Indiana UP, 1994.

Jones, Therese, Delese Wear, and Lester D. Friedman. "The Why, the What, and the How of the Medical/Health Humanities." *Health Humanities Reader.* Ed. Therese Jones, Delese Wear, and Lester D. Friedman. New Brunswick: Rutgers UP, 2014. 1–12.

Klass, Perri. "Breaking Gender Stereotypes in the Toy Box." *New York Times* 5 February 2018. www.nytimes.com/2018/02/05/well/family/gender-stereotypes-children-toys.html.

Scarry, Elaine. *The Body in Pain: The Making and Unmaking of the World.* Oxford: Oxford UP, 1985.

Spinner, Lauren. "Peer Toy Play as a Gateway to Children's Gender Flexibility: The Effect of (Counter)Stereotypic Portrayals of Peers in Children's Magazines." *Sex Roles* 79. 5–6 (September 2018): 314–328.

"Wheaties Commercial." 1978. www.yahoo.com/lifestyle/1978-flashback-bruce-jenner-wheaties-and-the-117171767386.html.

Zimmermann, Laura K. "Preschoolers' Perceptions of Gendered Toy Commercials in the US." *Journal of Children and Media* 11. 2(2017): 119–131.

Part I
Medical Models, Charts, and Institutional Narratives

2 Enlightened Wax Works

Viewing the Anatomical Woman in the Viennese Josephinum

Angelika Vybiral

Wax artifacts of anatomy were a popular instrument for anatomical studies in the eighteenth and nineteenth centuries in Europe. These devices were created as an alternative to real bodies. Wax models of the human body came into use over the course of the eighteenth century because they were a convenient replacement for corpses. Since opening human bodies was subject to religious and ethical taboos, anatomists began to create substitutes for human bodies. Wax served as the preferred material as it already had a long tradition in the production of relics, statues of saints, and votive offerings. This material was, therefore, part of contemporary representative art. Wax models often appeared more real than actual bodies because they preserved color and shape better. Additionally, anatomical wax models could be studied at any time and did not decay. They provided a more comfortable, cleaner, and more pleasant medium of transferring knowledge (Koblizek and Friedmann 89–92).

These models pretend to be realistic representations of nature and yet they do not have recourse to a real individualistic model but create a schematized image and show idealized nature. Around 1800, physicians directed their attention to the young, healthy, and beautiful body. Their representations exclude the repulsive qualities of the physical, the bodily fluids, and the misshapen. These wax models praise the idealized supra-individual beauty as God's creation: "Reality shall not be mirrored but shall become more recognizable in the wax model" (Almhofer 28).[1] Understanding the body was seen as understanding God; science could not be completely separated from religion. In the nineteenth century, the focus shifts to the pathologies of the body and therefore from aesthetics to naturalism (Lemire 92). Eighteenth-century wax models begin to be considered as "outdated scientific antiquarianism" (Krüger-Fürhoff 87), because they take an ideal and not reality as a model.

Making the Invisible Visible

Over the course of the eighteenth century, a radical epistemological change occurred within scientific discourse. Until then, anatomy was mainly taught using textbooks. Barbara Stafford labels this change a shift "from a text-based culture to a visually dependent culture" (xviii). We can understand this "visual turn" in science as a result of the Enlightenment, when Cartesian occularcentrism made vision the privileged sensory experience (Schwartz and Przyblyski 3–8). Science's aim to make the invisible visible is a modern approach. Such visualizing "has had some of its most dramatic effect in medicine, where everything [...] is now transformed into a visual pattern" (Mirzoeff 7). By lifting the veil—or in the case of anatomical wax models, the skin or the abdominal wall—the secrets of nature and truth are revealed and made visible. Viewing the body became part not only of medical education but also of public culture. The wax models allowed spectators to look under the skin of seemingly "living bodies" with their eyes and mouths half-opened. This anticipates what became possible only in the late nineteenth century with x-rays and was improved in twentieth-century medicine with new imaging techniques.

Gendered Anatomical Representations

Wax models belong simultaneously to the aesthetic, religious, and the scientific realms of eighteenth-century visual culture. Wax models imitate traditional forms of depicting the body in art and Christian modes of representation. Positioned between science and art, the models convey not only contemporary medical, but also cultural, ideas and ideals. They exemplify Enlightenment notions about the body and, from a perspective of gender, these wax models reveal connections between scientific materialism and cultural values. This chapter examines the gendered nature of female wax models and considers them as visual artifacts of the state of science and culture of the late eighteenth century. It is based on the assumption that science is intertwined with tacit knowledge and conveys ideas of culture and society by the means of the representation of knowledge. Strikingly, almost all female wax models of the eighteenth and nineteenth centuries are shown with skin, while skinned bodies are generally male. Discussing the cultural implications of female wax models by contrasting two models that are preserved in the historical-anatomical collection of the Medical University of Vienna, the Josephinum, this chapter analyzes the representation of women's bodies and the degree to which they confirm or clash with established gender norms.

The Institution and its Collection

The Josephinum was founded in 1785 by the Austrian Emperor Joseph II under the name of the Medical-Surgical Academy.[2] It was part of the largest public hospital in Europe at that time. Joseph II's prestige project embodied the ideas and values of Enlightenment absolutism (Horn and Lindenhofer 39). Worried by demographic concerns about a decline in both the number and the health of his population, the Emperor's aim was nothing less than to change Austrian society in its entirety. Health reforms aimed to strengthen the state's labor and armed forces. Since humans were considered a precious resource, policies regulating education, medicine, economy, and living conditions were introduced

(45–49). In this ambitious project, the Josephinum "was the central institution of a social concept meant to shape the future" (Horn 20). This academy was equipped with a comprehensive library collection, a morgue, a botanical garden, a wide range of medical instruments, and many other facilities. After his visit in 1780 to La Specola, the largest wax anatomical collection housed in the Museum of Natural History in Florence, Italy, Joseph II ordered copies of the 1,192 wax models in the La Specola collection to be included in his academy (Koblizek and Friedmann 92–97). They were reproduced in the workshop at La Specola in Florence between 1784 and 1788.[3] In line with Enlightenment ideals, the collection's purpose was not only to provide models for the medical training of future physicians but also to educate the public (Dacome 256). The anatomical wax models extended text-based knowledge by enabling haptic and visual and thus more immediate experiences while studying human anatomy. The wax models were and are still exhibited in rosewood cabinets behind Venetian glass that can be lifted to allow close inspection. Each model was accompanied by a watercolor drawing of the body/organ and a descriptive text. Originally, the collection contained two thousand wax models of which less than fifteen were full-body models, five of them female.[4]

The Josephinum's Female Full-Body Models

The collection includes five full-body female wax models. These are: MUW-0244 (Fig. 2.1), referred to as the *Mediceische Venus*, MUW-0245, and MUW-0190, all three in a recumbent position with their abdomens opened to show the womb and the intestines. Furthermore, there are two *écorchés:*[5] MUW-0060 (Fig. 2.2), an upright *écorché* and MUW-0125, a recumbent *écorché* lying on her stomach.[6] This study focuses on two of these models: the replication of the Florentine *Medici Venus* (MUW-0244), the so-called *Mediceische Venus*[7]—the most well-known wax model of the collection—and the female upright *écorché* (MUW-0060). These models represent two fundamentally different paradigms of depicting the anatomical woman: one with and one without skin.

The *Mediceische Venus* lies in a cabinet behind glass on white linen and lilac cushions. She is a copy of the famous wax model of the same name in the Florentine collection. The model displays a naked young woman with long blond hair, a pearl necklace, and a golden headband. Thick pubic hair covers her vulva. Her abdominal wall and her organs can be removed and reassembled like a modular system. In the Josephinum, she is displayed with her abdomen open; the removed parts are not displayed in the case. The removed parts reveal a pregnancy showing a five-month old fetus.

The second wax model is a female upright *écorché*. As *écorchés* are typically male, it is the only one of its kind in the anatomical wax collections in Europe.[8] This model stands out among the traditional forms of representation of female wax models as it adopts a posture that is usually associated with male models. *Écorchés* serve the study of the muscular system and the viscera by showing a flayed body. The description of this model (MUW-0060) tells us

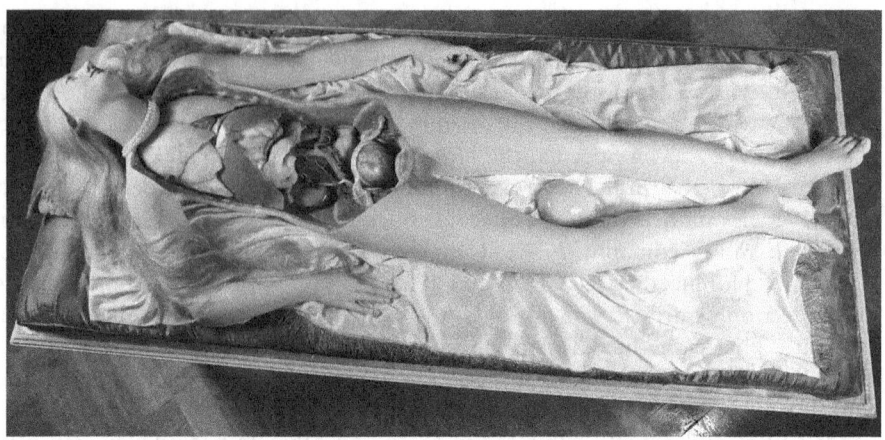

Figure 2.1 Mediceische Venus (MUW-0244). Courtesy of Josephinum—Ethik, Sammlungen und Geschichte der Medizin, MedUni Wien/Josephinum—Ethics,
   Collections and History of Medicine, MedUni Vienna

its purpose: "Female body: Representation of blood vessels, nerves, muscles
and intestines." The intestines are artificially arranged in order to allow a
view inside the body. The shell-like arrangement of the bowels can be interpreted as a metaphor for the intestinal convolutions, which are similarly
winding (Koblizek and Friedmann 88). *Écorchés* lack body hair because they
also lack skin. In contrast to male *écorchés*, however, this model has pubic
hair glued to its vulva; a detailed representation of the female sex is avoided
by hiding it under hair.

   Both the *Mediceische Venus* with her modular system and the *écorché* with
its removed skin are a metaphor for the anatomist's work: revealing and unco-
vering nature's secrets. The game of concealing and revealing uses a common
metaphor of the Enlightenment: Nature is personified as a woman, who is
hiding behind a veil that is lifted by the male scientist. This type of allegoric
representation can be found in the entrance hall of the medical school in Paris:
The sculpture *La nature se dévoilant devant la science* reflects the relationship
of female nature and male explorer that is part of the self-conception of science
in the Enlightenment.

Anatomical Craftsmanship between Art and Science

Both science and aesthetics played a major role in the creation of these models
(Dacome 253–254). Exhibited in a cabinet behind glass or, in the case of the
écorché, standing on a base, the spectator is kept at a distance. The elevated
position and the posture surround them with grandeur (Dürbeck 39). Anatomical wax models use established modes of representing ideal bodies. Their
aesthetic is derived from the canon of classical sculptures and Christian

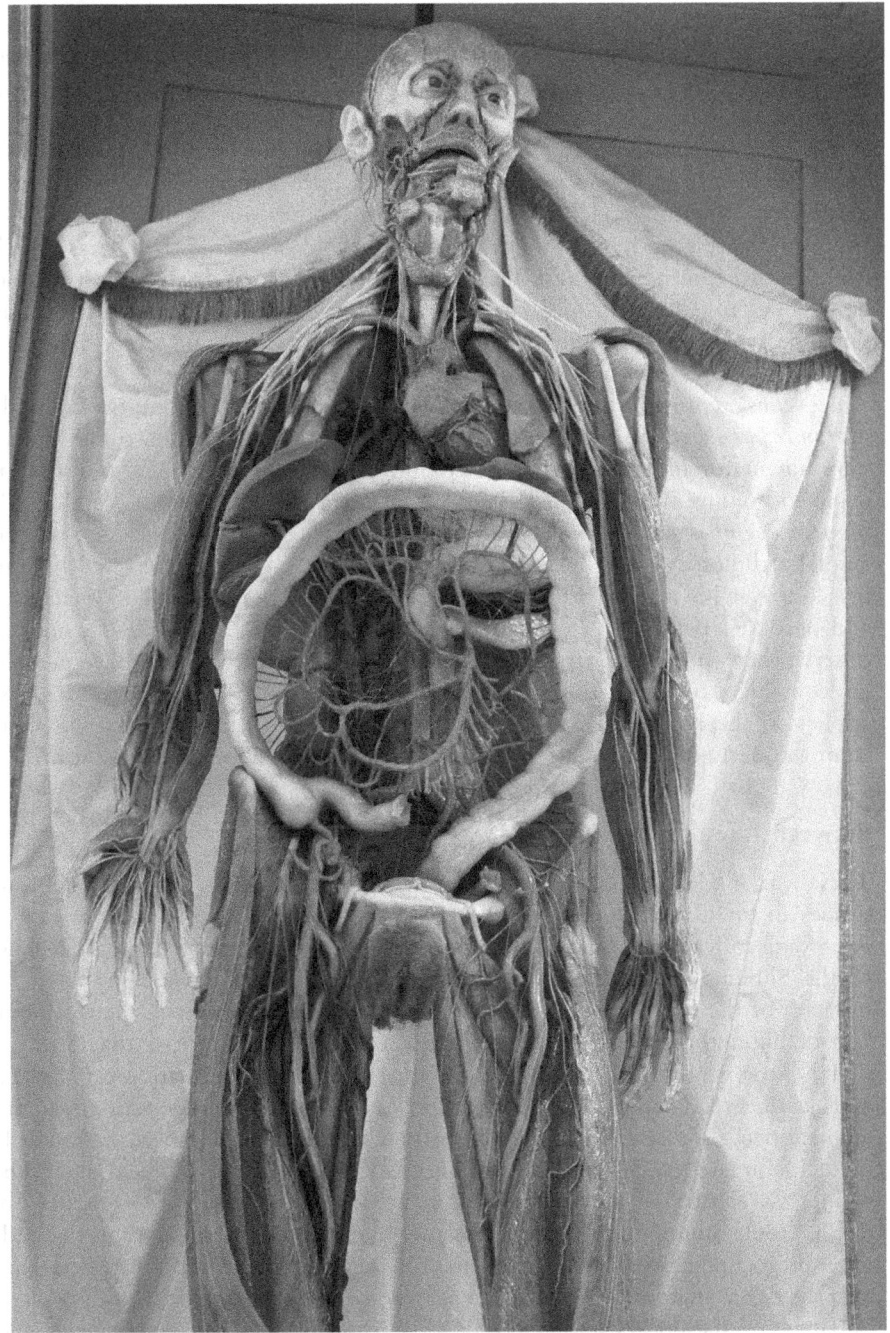

Figure 2.2 Female upright *écorché* (MUW-0060). Courtesy of Josephinum—Ethik,
Sammlungen und Geschichte der Medizin, MedUni Wien/Josephinum—
Ethics, Collections and History of Medicine, MedUni Vienna

iconography. Hartmut Böhme argues that echoing traditional ways of representation serves as a strategy of legitimization for the anatomist so as to render the bloody craft of anatomists more acceptable and appeal to spectators through familiarity (447).

Mediceische Venus refers to the ancient Roman goddess and to the sculpture of the same name. While numerous scholars have underlined the similarities between the antique model and the eighteenth-century wax figure (Dürbeck 47), the wax figure's body runs contrary to classic ideals of aesthetics, as Irmela Marei Krüger-Fürhoff argues: The wax model wears jewelry, the unity of her body is destroyed by the opening of the womb and her sex is highlighted by the pubic hair, which was omitted in classical art (93). Her name refers more to a well-known type than to actual similarities with her eponym.

Écorchés' representational meanings also originate from antiquity. In Ovid's *Metamorphosis* Marsyas was bound to a tree and skinned while still alive, as a punishment for his hubris towards Apollo. In artistic works, the *écorchés* are depicted holding their stripped skin over their arm like in Andrea Vesalius' *De humani corporis fabrica libri septum* (1543). In Christian iconography, we find Saint Bartholomew who was flayed as a martyr and is often depicted holding his skin over his arm.[9] Both served as an *exemplum doloris* in the Renaissance and Baroque (Benthien 97). Werner Telesko posits that, around 1800, one can observe that, in the fine arts, Enlightened clarity clashes with old Baroque allegories which continue to be omnipresent (178–182). This observation also applies to the representation of wax models. While their mise-en-scène stems from the Baroque, their educational impetus hails from the Enlightenment.

Between Life and Death

These wax models can be seen as examples of the "Sublime" that Immanuel Kant defines in his *Observations on the Feeling of the Beautiful and Sublime* (1764). According to Kant, the Sublime describes awe-inspiring greatness and the feelings of the Sublime "arouse enjoyment but with horror" (47). Contemplating the miracles of the body fills the observer with both horror and wonder, reminding him of his nothingness. It therefore does not come as a surprise that Sigmund Freud chose wax models as an example for the uncanny, oscillating between life and death. Freud writes that wax models cause "doubts whether an apparently animate being is really alive; or conversely, whether a lifeless object might not be in fact animate" (217). They simultaneously seem familiar and strange. This eeriness is caused by a cognitive dissonance exploring the borders of life and death. Contemplating the wax models provokes a voyeuristic shiver in the audience, or, as Francesco P. de Ceglia puts it, a "dizziness" (440). Both models—and also the other anatomical wax exhibits in the collection—cause this feeling of the Sublime and the uncanny for the following reasons: They cause both the fear of the inevitable death, functioning as memento mori, and the fear of the reduction of the human existence to a machine without soul. At the same time, however, the exclusion of the repulsive aspects of a corpse and the idealization of the body make death pleasant.

The two studied models achieve the balance between life and death differently. First, as Claudia Benthien (62) observes, the pearl necklace of the Medici Venus marks the division between the lively face and the opened trunk. The use of vivid colors, real hair, and the softness of the wax skin create the illusion of a human-like doll. While her open eyes and the half-opened mouth make her look animate, her divine name, "Venus," suggests immortality. Her passive posture, lying down full-length, and the fact that she can be taken apart make her look dead. Second, the skinned *écorché* conveys a degree of liveliness. Like male *écorchés*, her foot seems ready to walk, the half-opened mouth ready to talk. In contrast to her male counterparts, however, she does not extend one of her arms, making her appear less active. Both the *Mediceische Venus* and the female *écorché* are uncanny because they appear familiar and unfamiliar, being neither a corpse nor alive.

Between Abjection and Desire

Anatomical wax models excite the spectator's desire at the same time that they show the internal features of the body. While the *Mediceische Venus'* modular system visualizes the process of unveiling and penetrating the body, the *écorché* illustrates the result of this violent process because her skin has already been stripped off.

The *Mediceische Venus* highlights the sensuality and the beauty of the female body by an erotic process of visualization that plays with the morphology of the surface of the human body. The eroticized surface, the skin, is interrupted by the anatomical opening and discloses the inner secrets of the body. The process, or the imagined process, of removing the skin, of penetrating the body arouses the spectator. This opening means destruction. The desire to preserve the beautiful, perfect body opposes the desire to spoil, to open, to destroy (Didi-Huberman 108). The *Mediceische Venus'* ideal beauty in particular invites destruction and dismemberment, thereby mirroring two fascinations: Eros, the life instinct, and Thanatos, the death instinct, creating a "necro-erotic dissonance" (Böhme 465). The model evokes the fear of death and the dream of penetrating the body without consequence (Krüger-Fürhoff 89). The topos of female passivity has a strong erotic component and we can find it in the *Mediceische Venus'* posture. Feminist scholars like Mary Hunter point to the male physician's gaze at the dead wax woman, which subjects her to his fantasies and to his examination (43). The male spectator and his hands find a defenseless, naked, immobile body that he can disassemble, destroy, and reassemble at his pleasure. The *Venus* takes a passive position as she turns away her head "as if she were offering herself up for sacrifice to an unknown torturer without daring to look at him" (de Ceglia 437). These erotic connotations are stressed by the staging of the *Mediceische Venus* on a silken bed and the pearls around her neck, which are a symbol for seduction and love. Joanna Ebenstein (180–186) by contrast interprets the *Venus'* look into the void as an ecstatic mystical experience. Her look is comparable to the High Baroque depiction of Saint Teresa, which can be found in the statue of the same name by Gian Lorenzo Bernini shown in a chapel in the church Santa Maria della Vittoria in Rome.

The *écorché*, on the other hand is barely recognizable as a woman. Only taking a closer look at the sex reveals that it is a female model. It lacks eroticism and breaks the taboo of the skinned woman, as Claudia Benthien (97–101) notices. Showing the layers in-between threatens the order of desire. The skinned woman is not a woman anymore. She can only be feminine on her surface, the skin, or as a container, showing her womb, but not without the covering shell. Thereby the *écorché*, representing mainly an intellectual approach, excites only the desire to know and not an erotic desire. The *écorché* is solely horrific, whereas the *Venus'* idealized beautiful outside is erotic and only her *inside* is horrific. In this sense, unlike the *écorché*, the *Mediceische Venus* and the models MUW-0245 and MUW-0190 correspond to the typical eighteenth-century representation of femininity. These models exude eroticism through their pose, their long hair, their half-opened eyes, and their accented lips. What unites the *Mediceische Venus*, MUW-0245 and MUW-0190 is the fact of having skin, which is the surface of eroticism and femininity.

Skin-Deep Femininity

In eighteenth-century medicine, the skin as the organ of sensibility was connoted as female and the muscles as male (Jordanova 58). Claudia Benthien observes that the "encoding of femininity takes place on the skin, the one of masculinity underneath" (100). The woman is a woman on her skin and in her inner (reproductive) organs (Benthien 97–98). A common metaphor for the female body since antiquity is the vessel; this explains the focus on the womb, the reproductive, and the intestinal organs.[10] The skinning of a woman is a taboo and therefore female *écorchés* showing the muscular, nervous or lymphatic system are very rare. The surface or the innermost parts of the female body are examined but rarely the layers in between. They are seen as a wound, as obscene, ugly, bloody, and diffuse. The female skin is a concealing veil, hence removing it destroys the myth of the woman's otherness. Only the muddy inner—especially the reproductive organs of the body—or the exterior surface—the immaculate skin—make a female, not the in-between such as the muscles or nerves. The woman is the surface and container at the same time, as Benthien (98–101) describes it. Therefore, the skin as a symbol of sensualism and sensuality is a female attribute of wax models. The Josephinum's female *écorché* seems to be an exception and questions the traditional representation of anatomical women.[11] Traditional representations, like the *Mediceische Venus*, emphasize the reproductive potential of the female body,[12] mirroring normative descriptions of women's role in society in such publications as the *Encyclopédie*.

Conclusion

In the Enlightenment concept of femininity, the woman is spouse und mother. She is pious, loving, gentle, pure, sensitive, and caring, as we can read in the French *Encyclopédie* in the article "femme (morale)" (Desmahis 472–475). In medicine, the male body is conceived as the standard human body type and the female as a deviant form, primarily utilized to portray reproduction and birth. Claudia Honegger labels this representation the "weibliche Sonderanthropologie" [female special anthropology] and locates its origin in the eighteenth century. This anthropology depicts fundamental differences between the sexes that were first conceptualized in literature and philosophy and later naturalized through science (Honegger 165). Around 1800, physicians localized sex differences in every organ, bone, muscle, and fiber.[13] The differences were deterministically attributed to motherhood, and led to the naturalized role of the woman in family and society (Schiebinger 42–43). These cultural and scientific perceptions shaped the medicalized visual and moral representation of the female wax models and found their way into anatomical illustrations of the body. The majority of wax models in the Viennese Medical-Surgical Academy focus on generation and birth. Even though the upright female *écorché* depicts the womb, it also shows the muscular, the nervous, the lymphatic, and the blood systems, like its male counterpart. The female upright *écorché* challenges eighteenth-century gender norms through its mere existence, yet it is still bound by them. The focus remains on the womb and the posture differs from that of male *écorchés*. While male *écorchés* stretch out one arm, this female figure has a rather reserved posture with its arms close to its body. The male *écorchés* lift one foot in the classical contrapposto manner. By contrast, females are bound to the ground with both feet firmly standing on the base in the case of MUW-060 or lying down on her abdomen in MUW-0125. Both postures emphasize female passivity. Skin also functions as a signifier of femininity around 1800.[14] The absence of skin questions traditional representations of femininity and could explain why this kind of model is rare in anatomical collections of the time.

Notes

1 All translations are mine, unless otherwise noted.
2 It was officially named "Josephs-Academie" or "Collegium-Medico-Chirurgicum-Josephinum" and was abbreviated as "Josephinum." On the history and the collection of the Josephinum, see Gröger and Horn and Ablogin.
3 The original Anatomical Venus was produced by Clemente Susini between 1780 and 1782 in Florence, Italy.
4 The others depicted specific muscles, organs, parts of the nervous system, or fetuses in different stages of development.
5 An *écorché* is a flayed body and the term used to describe the representation of a skinned body for anatomical studies. It is the past participle of the French verb "écorcher," which means "to skin, to flay."
6 There are also partial models representing specific female body parts such as the uterus and the clitoris.

7   Its full name is *Eine Nachbildung der Mediceischen Venus; mit herausnehmbaren Eingeweiden*, MUW-0244 (Allmer and Jantsch 70).
8   It is the only one to my knowledge. There might be another female upright *écorché* in London but I have not yet had the chance to verify this information.
9   See for example, Camillo Rusconi's statue of Saint Bartholomew from 1715, which is located in the Basilica San Giovanni in Laterano in Rome. In the Dome of Milan, Marco d'Agrate's statue (1542) shows the saint carrying his skin wrapped around his shoulders. In the Sistine Chapel, Bartholomew is depicted holding his skin in his hand.
10 Still there is no explanation of the representation of the model MUW-0125, which shows neither reproductive organs nor intestines.
11 The other female *écorché* in the Josephinum (MUW-0125) comes closer to typical representational modes of women, even though she is shown without skin, because she is displayed in a recumbent passive position, lying on her abdomen.
12 See in particular the extensive obstetric collection in Allmer and Jantsch 66–69, 90–96.
13 Pierre Roussel's *Système physique et moral de la femme* (1775) is considered a founding text for the moral-medical philosophy on women.
14 This observation applies to other exhibits in the collection. Those who show an arm or a hand with skin often depict feminine hands.

Works Cited

Allmer, Konrad and Marlene Jantsch. *Katalog der Josephinischen Sammlung an der Universität Wien*. Cologne: Böhlau, 1965.

Almhofer, Edith. "Beredte Bilder des Leibes." *Anatomie als Kunst: Anatomische Wachsmodelle des 18. Jahrhunderts im Josephinum in Wien*. Ed. M. Skopec et al. Vienna: Brandstätter, 2002. 21–29.

Benthien, Claudia. *Haut. Literaturgeschichte, Körperbilder, Grenzdiskurse*. Reinbek bei Hamburg: Rowohlt Taschenbuch, 1999.

Bergmann, Anna. "Die Verlebendigung des Todes und die Tötung des Lebendigen durch den medizinischen Blick." *Körper—Geschlecht—Geschichte: Historische und aktuelle Debatten in der Medizin*. Ed. E. Mixa. Innsbruck: Studienverlag, 1996. 77–95.

Böhme, Hartmut. "Nacktheit und Scham in der Anatomie der Frühen Neuzeit." *Scham und Schamhaftigkeit: Grenzverletzungen in Literatur und Kultur der Vormoderne*. Ed. Katja Gvozdeva and Hans Rudolf Velten. Berlin: de Gruyter, 2011. 434–470.

Dacome, Lucia. "Inszenierung des Körpers: Anatomische Wachsplastik im Zeitalter Mozarts. Ein neues Lehrmitte der Anatomie." *Mozart: Experiment Aufklärung im Wien des ausgehenden 18. Jahrhunderts*. Ed. Herbert Lachmayer. Vienna: Hatje Cantz, 2008. 249–259.

De Ceglia, Francesco Paolo. "Rotten Corpses, a Disembowelled Woman, a Flayed Man: Images of the Body from the End of the 17th to the Beginning of the 19th Century. Florentine Wax Models in the First-hand Accounts of Visitors." *Perspectives on Science* 14. 4(2006): 417–456.

Desmahis, Jean-François-Edouard de Corsembleu de. "Femme (Morale)." *Encyclopédie, ou dictionnaire raisonné des sciences, des arts et des métiers, par une société de gens de lettres*. Ed. D. Diderot and J.B. le Rond d'Alembert. Paris, 1756. Vol. VI. 472–475.

Didi-Huberman, Georges. *Venus öffnen: Nacktheit, Traum, Grausamkeit*. Zurich: Diaphanes, 2006.

Dürbeck, Gabriele. "Empirischer und ästhetischer Sinn: Strategien der Vermittlung von Wissen in der anatomischen Wachsplastik um 1780." *Wahrnehmung der Natur: Natur der Wahrnehmung. Studien zur Geschichte visueller Kultur um 1800*. Ed. Gabriele Dürbeck et al. Dresden: Verlag der Kunst, 2001. 35–54.

Ebenstein, Joanna. *The Anatomical Venus*. London: Thames & Hudson, 2016.

Freud, Sigmund. "The Uncanny." *The Standard Edition of the Complete Psychological Works of Sigmund Freud*. Vol. XVII. Trans. and ed. J. Strachey et al. London: Hogarth, 1955. 217–256.

Gröger, Helmut. "Die Gründung der medizinisch-chirurgischen Josephs-Akademie und ihre Sammlung anatomischer Wachspräparate." *Mozart: Experiment Aufklärung im Wien des ausgehenden 18. Jahrhunderts*. Ed. Herbert Lachmayer. Vienna: Hatje Cantz, 2006. 241–248.

Honegger, Claudia. *Die Ordnung der Geschlechter: Die Wissenschaften vom Menschen und vom Weib 1750–1850*. Frankfurt am Main: Campus Verlag, 1991.

Horn, Sonia. "Einleitung." *Faszination Josephinum: Die anatomischen Wachspräparate und ihr Haus*. Ed. Sonia Horn and Alexander Ablogin. Vienna: Verlagshaus der Ärzte, 2012. 11–22.

Horn, Sonia and Alexander Ablogin, eds. *Faszination Josephinum: Die anatomischen Wachspräparate und ihr Haus*. Vienna: Verlagshaus der Ärzte, 2012.

Horn, Sonia and Petra Lindenhofer. "Das Josephinum—Eine Institution im gesundheitspolitischen und wirtschaftlichen Kontext des 18. Jahrhunderts." *Faszination Josephinum. Die anatomischen Wachspräparate und ihr Haus*. Ed. Sonia. Horn and Alexander Ablogin. Vienna: Verlagshaus der Ärzte, 2012. 23–50.

Hunter, Mary. "Effroyable réalisme: Wax, Femininity, and the Madness of Realist Fantasies." *Revue d'art canadienne/Canadian Art Review* 33. 1–2(2008): 43–58.

Jordanova, Ludmilla. *Sexual Visions: Images of Gender in Science and Medicine between the Eighteenth and Twentieth Centuries*. Madison: U of Wisconsin P, 1989.

Kant, Immanuel. *Observations on the Feeling of the Beautiful and Sublime*. Trans. J.T. Goldthwait. Berkeley: U of California P, 1965.

Koblizek, Ruth and Ina Friedmann. "Kunst und Anatomie im 18. Jahrhundert." *Faszination Josephinum: Die anatomischen Wachspräparate und ihr Haus*. Ed. Sonia Horn and Alexander Ablogin. Vienna: Verlagshaus der Ärzte, 2012. 85–114.

Krüger-Fürhoff, Irmela M. *Der versehrte Körper. Revisionen des klassizistischen Schönheitsideals*. Göttingen: Wallstein, 2001.

Lemire, Michel. "Fortunes et infortunes de l'anatomie et des préparations anatomiques, naturelles et artificielles." *L'âme au corps. Arts et science 1793–1993, Catalogue. Galéries nationales du Grand Palais 19 octobre 1993–24 janvier 1994*. Ed. J. Clair. Paris: Gallimard/Electa, 1993. 70–101.

Mirzoeff, Nicholas. "What Is Visual Culture?" *The Visual Culture Reader*. Ed. Nicholas Mirzoeff. London: Routledge, 1998. 3–13.

Schiebinger, Londa. "Skeletons in the Closet: The First Illustrations of the Female Skeleton in Eighteenth-Century Anatomy." *Representations* 14(1986): 42–82.

Schwartz, Vanessa R. and Jeannene M. Przyblyski. "Visual Culture's History. Twenty-first Century Interdisciplinarity and its Nineteenth-Century Objects." *The Nineteenth-Century Visual Culture Reader*. Ed. Vanessa R. Schwartz and Jeannene M. Przyblyski. New York: Routledge, 2004. 3–14.

Stafford, Barbara Maria. *Body Criticism: Imagining the Unseen in Enlightenment Art and Medicine*. Cambridge: MIT Press, 1991.

Telesko, Werner. *Einführung in die Ikonographie der barocken Kunst*. Cologne: Böhlau, 2005.

3 Epistemological Anxiety
The Case of Michel-Anne Drouart

Stephanie M. Hilger

Sexually ambiguous bodies have occupied the human imagination since antiquity, with early writings often invoking the nymph Salmacis, whose love for Hermaphroditus made her fuse their forms, creating a two-sexed human. By the late seventeenth century, however, writings on hermaphrodites[1] distanced themselves from mythology, striving instead for scientific explanations. While much scholarship on hermaphroditism focuses on the nineteenth century,[2] the modern understanding of what is now called intersexuality originated in the eighteenth century. Londa Schiebinger argues that this period:

> saw the emergence of modern science, (what we have come to call) scientific sexism related to modern notions of femininity and masculinity, and scientific racism. This triad—science, and scientific notions of sexual and racial differences—emerged not as disassociated and unencumbered phenomena, but as developments that formed each other in decisive ways.
>
> (*Nature's Body* xi)

The eighteenth century marks a pivotal moment in scientific endeavors to understand hermaphrodites, and these ambiguous bodies are inextricably intertwined with evolving notions of gender and race as well as developments in the scientific and political realms.

Intense scrutiny of hermaphrodites mirrors a new focus on the individual:

> As individual bodies came to take a central place within an economic, intellectual, moral, and political order, bodies were increasingly scrutinized for marks of difference that might give a clue to a person's, or class of persons', place in that order.
>
> (Schiebinger, *Nature's Body* xii)

The hermaphroditic body abounded with marks of difference, creating an investigational object *par excellence*. Scientific and medical inquiries sought to erase ambiguity, wielding the tools of Enlightenment science to classify such bodies as male or female.

Narrative Constructions and Epistemological Shifts

While the genre of the case study had existed since Hippocrates, its production accelerated in the eighteenth century because it supported an increased focus on the individual as well as empiricism. Case studies by medical and legal experts informed court decisions on the official sex of ambiguous individuals and could have serious consequences for inheritance and marriage. These case studies also circulated to a wide readership, which was made possible by the use of the vernacular rather than Latin.[3] Many case studies on hermaphroditic bodies became bestsellers, some as popular as novels, with which they share the focus on one individual in unusual or extreme circumstances.

Traditional scholarship on eighteenth-century case studies on hermaphrodites largely follows Michel Foucault's *Les anormaux* (1974–1975), which posits that these studies deny sexual ambivalence by classifying bodies as either male or female.[4] Thus, Enlightenment accounts are seen as the first step in moving ambiguously sexed bodies from mythology to the scientific/medical realm.[5] This reading, however, obscures the fact that these studies are marked by intellectual anxiety caused by profound epistemological shifts during the Enlightenment, resulting in the rise and popularization of empirical science, competing theories of generation and female sexual pleasure, and the professionalization of medicine. This intellectual anxiety crystallizes in attempts to control and classify the hermaphroditic body, which became a symbol of the changes to centuries-old ways of knowing. Yet the hermaphroditic body thwarted scientific efforts to elucidate its workings. A literary-critical reading of these case studies, which blur the line between science and literature, uncovers this epistemological anxiety by investigating narrative structures and discursive techniques that construct, rather than simply describe, hermaphroditic bodies.

Michel-Anne Drouart, the Hermaphrodite

One of the most famous hermaphrodites was Michel-Anne Drouart, born to parents of modest means in Paris in 1733 and raised as a girl. The Drouart home was visited by the curious as news of Michel-Anne's unusual genitalia spread. Although authorities at the Sorbonne declared Drouart male, doubts persisted. Drouart was eventually sent to a London surgeon who exhibited him for a fee. Drouart then traveled throughout Europe, displaying his body to various medical professionals. Their exams became the basis for a dense textual web of publications, which made Drouart a celebrity well beyond the medical realm.

The main publications by M. Mertrud (1749), Sauveur Francois Morand (1749), M. Vacherie (1750), D. Gottfried Heinrich Burghart (1763), Heinrich Friederich Delius (1765), Antoine Ferrein (1767), and Jean Jacques Louis Hoin (1761) come to diametrically opposed conclusions regarding Drouart's sex. However, these authors all share similar anxieties about securing their place in the scientific realm during profound epistemological changes. My analysis does not purport to solve the riddle of Drouart's body but investigates the unstable epistemological terrain these authors navigated in examining the hermaphroditic physique.

Empiricism

The first publication on Drouart is M. Mertrud's 1749 *Hermaphrodite, dissertation au sujet de la fameuse hermaphrodite qui a paru aux yeux du public depuis environ trois mois* [Hermaphrodite, dissertation on the subject of the famous hermaphrodite who has been appearing in front of the public for approximately three months].[6] Mertrud positions himself strategically as the "full-time royal surgeon, sworn in at St Côme by the Academy and anatomical and surgical demonstrator at King's Garden [the natural history museum]" ["chirurgien ordinaire du roi, juré à St Côme, de son Académie, et démonstrateur en anatomie et chirurgie au jardin du roi"] (n.p.), establishing his connection to traditional structures of knowledge production by highlighting his position at court. He also identifies himself as a surgeon and anatomical demonstrator, which is significant in the context of the rising demand for empirical knowledge of the human body. The first half of Mertrud's text provides a detailed description of Drouart's genitals and references the accompanying two-page illustration by Jacques-Fabien Gautier d'Agoty, an engraver working in the king's service. At the time, Drouart was sixteen years old and Mertrud concluded that a dominant sex would emerge after puberty, thereby opening the door to sequels. For Mertrud, Drouart is only seemingly a hermaphrodite or "pseudo-hermaphrodite," whom eighteenth-century scholarship could classify as male, female, or as a variation in which neither sex dominated. While Mertrud avoids explicit pronouncements regarding Drouart's sex, his use of the female grammatical gender acknowledges the sex in which Drouart was raised and may function as an unconscious revelation of Mertrud's beliefs.[7] Mertrud transformed Drouart into a veritable celebrity. Mertrud's *Dissertation* was republished in Volume I of the *Journal de physique* (1752) (Graille 222) and became the first chapter in Drouart's story.

At the same time that Mertrud subscribes to the increasing demand for empirical science—he examines Drouart, describes the genitals in detail, and appends an illustration—his scientific frame of reference remains rooted in the past. In the second part of his text, he discusses the Greek myth of Hermaphroditus, summarizes Ovid's account, and references seventeenth- and eighteenth-century authors on the topic. Mertrud thereby invokes the predominant pre-eighteenth-century mode of knowledge production, which mainly consisted of lengthy summaries and commentaries on previously produced writings, going back to Antiquity, typically without any first-hand scientific investigation.[8] Mertrud appears to be ambivalent about the epistemological shift towards empiricism; later publications, however, all distance themselves from mythologically based explanations of this phenomenon.

Another empirical text, Sauveur-François Morand's *Description d'un hermaphrodite, que l'on voyait à Paris en 1749* [Description of a hermaphrodite seen in Paris in 1749] appeared in the *Mémoires de l'Académie Royale des Sciences de Paris* in 1750 and was republished in Jean-Michel Moreau's *Garçon et fille hermaphrodites vus et dessinés d'après nature* [Hermaphroditic boy and girl viewed and drawn according to nature] (1773), accompanied by two illustrations. Famous for the removal of kidney stones, Morand was one of Paris' premier surgeons. In 1743, he published *Discours dans lequel on prouve qu'il est néces-saire au chirurgien d'être lettré* [Treatise in which it is proven that a surgeon needs to be lettered], arguing that surgeons needed general medical knowledge, literacy in classical languages, logic, and physics, to become *lettré*, lettered gen-tlemen, like their physician competitors. His treatise contributed to the pamphlet warfare between physicians and surgeons in 1730s and 1740s Paris, from which surgeons emerged victorious with royal decrees in 1740 and 1750. As a specialist of the urogenital system and demonstrator of surgery at the *Jardin du Roi*, a crown-supported surgical theater, Morand's publications about Drouart served a strategic function; they allowed him to highlight his connection to the political status quo and his position in the emerging medical marketplace.[9]

Rumors about a living hermaphrodite led Morand to examine Drouart. Unlike Mertrud, Morand never invokes the Greek myth of Hermaphroditus; he instead provides the reader with a detailed account of Drouart's genitals and argues that, despite "a strange mixture of both sexes" ["une sorte de mélange bizarre des deux Sexes"] (4), "the masculine sex dominates" ["le sexe masculin domine"] (4). He emphasizes his aim to "keep to a simple description of the parts" ["[j]e me tiens à la simple description des parties"] and his role as "observer" ["observateur"] (4). Thus, Morand marshals empiricism in the service of objectivity rather than moral judgment.

Popular Science

A year later, M. Vacherie, a Brussels surgeon, performed his own exam of Drouart, producing a more extensive description than either Mertrud or Morand. Vacherie presents his account for the benefit of those who were unable to see Drouart at all or in his fullest maturity, establishing a link to Mertrud's text. Vacherie's title page positions his treatise for a broad audience and, in the manner of popular broadsides, caters to readers' voyeurism: "An Account of the Famous Hermaphrodite, or, Parisian Boy-Girl, aged Sixteen, named Michael-Anne Drouart, At This Time (November, 1750) upon Show in Car-naby-Street, London. With its Portrait Engraved from the Life." Describing Drouart as the "Parisian Boy-Girl" situates Vacherie's text among popular-sci-entific treatises of the period. Like his predecessors, Vacherie underlines his role as observer, striving to uncover what is hidden from view. He also notes that he "sprea[d] the thighs" (10) and his "exploring touch" (11) allowed him to "soun [d] deeper in" (11) than those preceding him. The emphasis on empirical method, thus, also caters to audience voyeurism, blurring the line between sci-entific and erotic/pornographic discourse.[10] Vacherie's identification of Drouart as a "boy-girl" produces salacious reading material even as it expresses his inability to determine Drouart's sex. In fact, consistent use of the pronoun "it" acknowledges the existence of a being that frustrates Vacherie's empiricism.

Reproduction and Sexual Pleasure

A most fascinating question for Enlightenment scientists was the reproductive potential of the hermaphrodite. Like hermaphroditic invertebrates such as slugs and worms, true human hermaphrodites were thought to have the capacity for self-fertilization. Therefore, hermaphrodites were part of broader debates on human reproduction. Scientists studying reproduction in the seventeenth and eighteenth centuries can be divided into two main groups, preformationists and epigenesists. Preformationists believed that a miniature human (homunculus) existed preformed either in the female egg or male sperm. By contrast, epigenesists believed that the fetus arose from the merging of two fluids. Considerable difficulties emerged in proving and defending either theory. At the same time, the role of clitoral orgasm in reproduction, thought analogous to ejaculation in the seventeenth century, became increasingly threatening because it called male superiority into question. As a result, clitoral pleasure became pathologized, a topic worthy of discussion only in the context of malformation.[11]

While Mertrud's and Vacherie's anatomical descriptions do not address Drouart's sensations, Morand and Jean Jacques Louis Hoin, writing in 1761 both thematize this question. In support of his thesis that Drouart is more masculine, Morand emphasizes his subject's erections: "upon waking up, the hermaphrodite sometimes experiences a more or less powerful erection that can last for an entire hour" ["l'Hermaphrodite a souvent à son réveil, de l'érection plus ou moins forte, qui se soutient environ une heure de suite"] ("Description" 3–4). When Drouart's seemingly female genitals do not respond to the male scientist's exploratory advances, Morand concludes that Drouart must be a man: "He does not at all respond to the insertion of the finger into the feminine part, not even to the movements made to excite him" ["Il n'est point du tout sensible à l'introduction du doigt dans la partie feminine, même aux mouvemens que l'on feroit pour l'exciter"] (4).

In Jean Jacques Louis Hoin's *Nouvelle Description de l'Hermaphrodite Drouart* [New Description of the Hermaphrodite Drouart], originally published on its own in 1761 and then republished as part of the *Mémoires de l'Académie de Dijon* in 1772, the issue of sexual pleasure is more complex. Hoin comes to a different conclusion when he describes the "erection with which we surprised her once" ["érection où nous l'avons surprise une fois"] (3). The grammatical construction, "surprise," is feminine, indicating that, for Hoin, Drouart is a woman.[12] While he does not use the word clitoris, Hoin considers the anatomical organ that resembles a penis to function as one, as in his description of Drouart's daydreaming: "a half-voluptuous awakening that caused the natural excretion of a limpid humor in her vagina ["un réveil à demi voluptueux, en occasionnant dans son vagin l'excrétion naturelle d'une humeur limpide"] (7). This phrase points at the persisting analogy beteen clitoral and penile orgasm and also appeals to the audience's voyeuristic desire: Drouart is caught having an erection by the ever-observing scientist and, hence, the reader. Hoin concludes that Drouart could not sire children but, with surgery to open the entrance to the vagina, might be able to bear them:

we do not risk anything by assuring you that the masculine part would be absolutely unsuitable for generation ... he hoped to become a mother; we do not see anything that would prevent him from becoming one after having undergone the proposed operation.

[nous ne hazardons rien en assurant que la partie masculine seroit absolument impropre à la génération ... il espéroit devenir mère; qualité que nous ne voyons rien qui puisse l'empêcher d'acquérir physiquement, après qu'il auroit souffert l'opération proposée].

(7)

Despite this conclusion, however, Hoin continues to refer to Drouart as "he," resulting in the paradoxical phrase "he hoped to become a mother" ["il espéroit devenir mère"]. While Hoin appears to respect Drouart's decision to live as a man, these ambivalent phrases point at Hoin's desire to rewrite Drouart's story and become its hero by surgically normalizing malfunctioning genitalia.

Changes in the Medical Profession

Surgeons Mertrud, Morand, Hoin, and Vacherie all publish against the backdrop of significant changes in the medical profession and education. The training and education of surgeons mainly occurred in the context of an apprenticeship. Therefore, as Roy Porter observes, surgery was considered "a manual skill rather than a liberal science" (277). By contrast, physicians were considered gentlemen, trained at university and licensed by professional associations. Whereas surgical training emphasized practical knowledge, academic medical education focused on reviewing and evaluating knowledge published since antiquity. During the eighteenth century, the separation between surgeons and physicians began to erode, leading to what Thomas Neville Bonner calls a "rapprochement" (56).[13] Surgeons gradually separated from barbers, creating professional associations and attending courses at private medical schools or hospitals. Likewise, university-trained physicians, who mainly possessed theoretical knowledge, increasingly began to participate in anatomical dissections; empirical knowledge was destigmatized and became positive currency in the medical field.

Publishing a case study that garnered significant attention was a way of establishing and consolidating the author's professional standing in a medical marketplace where he was competing with a broad range of "unincorporated healers [such as] toothpullers, wise women, patent remedy vendors, herbalists, pedlars, diviners, astrologers, and faith healers" (Spary 84). In England, individual entrepreneurship was stronger than in France, where the corporative system of professional organizations continued to exert influence throughout the eighteenth century, or in the German-speaking territories, where universities were more closely involved in surgical training. Vacherie's advertisement of his text in the manner of popular broadsides in the London medical marketplace is indicative in this respect. Those publishing in France typically foregrounded their membership in national or regional professional associations, which were connected to royal authority in pre-Revolutionary times. Thus Mertrud identifies himself as the "full-time royal surgeon" ["chirurgien ordinaire du roi"]. Similarly, Morand demonstrated surgery at a crown-supported surgical theater, and Hoin was a member of the *Académie de Dijon* and the *Académie royale de chirurgie*. Publishing a sensational case story on a hermaphrodite was a way of adapting to a quickly changing professional environment, in which individual entrepreneurship threatened medical authorities' privileged status.

Science and Power

Significant changes in medical training in German-speaking lands occurred during the reign of Frederick Wilhelm I (1688–1740) and Frederick the Great (1740–1786). Medicine was practical, improving treatment of battlefield wounds as well as that of the general population. In 1725, the *collegium medico-chirurgicum* was created, its operation intertwined with instruction at the *theatrum anatomicum* and "integrated with the 'learned' or university-based prestige of the internist" (Geyer-Kordesch 204). The *collegium medicum* in Berlin enforced its power through a network of regulations. Frederick the Great continued his father's legacy by emphasizing medicine's role in public health and maintaining the strength of the Prussian state.[14] Unlike his father, Frederick II filled important positions in his medical administration with Frenchmen (Geyer-Kordesch 204).

During Frederick the Great's reign, anxiety about the medical profession and its connection to political power surfaced in a little-known German description of Drouart, D. Gottfried Heinrich Burghart's 1763 *Gründliche Nachricht an seinen Freund *** Von einem neuerlich gesehenen Hermaphroditen, Wobey zugleich etwas von der Medicinischen Mode erwähnet wird* [Detailed Account to his Friend *** regarding a recently examined hermaphrodite, to which is added a discussion of medical fashion]. Only one-third of the twenty-four-page text directly discusses Drouart, whose case follows Burghart's reflections on the medical profession. Burghart emphasizes his position in a Prussian educational institution, its connection to the ruler, and his membership in various learned societies when he identifies himself as "medical professor and full-time teacher of mathematics and natural sciences at the royal college in Brieg, the imperial academy of natural scientists ... and a member of the imperial-royal society of belles lettres" ["Med. Professoris Primarii und ordentlichen offentlichen Lehrers der Mathematik und Naturkunde am Königl. Collegio zu Brieg, der Kaiserl. Reichs- Academie der Naturforscher ... Und der Kaiserl. Königl. Gesellschaft der schönen Wissenschaften Mitglieds"]. He makes a lengthy dedication to Frederick the Great, presenting himself as a loyal subject:

> As I am convinced of your highness' liking of me, the small amount of fear that my writing and the news in it that is meant for you, will be received unfavorably, will be sufficient. ... I am now writing without fear because I do not have the impression to displease you.

[Wie sehr ich von Ewr. Hochedlgeb. Schätzbaren neigung gegen mich überzeugt sei, wird die wenige Furcht, daß mein Schreiben und die Ihnen darinnen bestimmte Neuigkeit ungütig aufgenommen werden möchte, zu Genüge darthun ... Ich schreibe also jetzt ohne Furcht, weil mich keine Vermuthung zu mißfallen zurücke hält ...].

(3)

Brieg, formerly Austrian, had become part of Prussia in 1741, and Burghart writes at the end of the Seven Years' War (1756–1763), in which Britain and Prussia defeated France and Austria.

Believing that Drouart is more likely to bear than engender a child, Burghart considers the Sorbonne's determination that Drouart was male to be "ridiculous" ["lächerlich"] (21). Burghart's case study also presents a broader critique of the supremacy of French language, culture, and intellectual production. He mocks the "fashionable doctor" ["Mode-Arzt"] who diagnoses "a languishing air (French again)" ["ein Air languisant (abermals französisch)"] (13), a typical criticism by European contemporaries who feared that the seeming feminization of French men would spread across the continent: "Dear young men, do not think that the latest fashion in medicine only affects the fair sex and lets you escape" ["Denket ja nicht ihr lieben jungen Herrn! daß die Arzneikunst nach der Mode, nur bloß das schöne Geschlecht antaste, und euch ungerupft durchwischen lasse"] (13). Thus Burghart implicitly reinforces the masculinity of the Anglo-Prussian coalition, which questioned French supremacy and significantly shifted power dynamics. Yet, while these comments flattered the Prussian status quo, they were potentially hazardous as attacks on Frederick II's francophilia, which manifested in his appointment of French physicians to the Prussian medical establishment.

In line with his self-presentation as an old-fashioned doctor, Burghart ridicules new methods of medical training:

> a few years at an institution of higher learning now create a real artist after the new fashion. A little bit of mathematics, a dissected human body, a few strangled human dogs, some observed chemical experiments, an air pump that has been touched three times, and finally a bag full of metaphysical truths.
>
> [ein paar Jahre Zeit auf der Hohen Schule bilden einen ächten Künstler nach der neuen Mode. Ein bißgen Mathematik, ein zerschnittner menschlicher Cörper, ein Paar erwürgte Hunde, etliche gesehene Chemische Versuche, eine dreimahl angerührte Lufftpumpe, und endlich ein Sackvoll metaphysischer Wahrheiten].

(5)

He criticizes both those who immerse themselves in books and those who acquire knowledge through dissections. Instead, Burghart values old-fashioned physicians like himself who spend time at their patients' bedside and develop "practical medicine" ["praktische Heilkunst"] (14) based on "accurate observations, reliable experiences ... as possibilities of explanation" ["genaue Beobachtungen, sichere Erfahrungen ... [als] Möglichkeit der Erklärungen"] (9).

By presenting himself as a mature physician-citizen, Burghart positions himself as a mentor while indirectly expressing fear of being replaced by a French colleague. By engaging one of the most vigorously debated phenomena in the medical field, hermaphroditism, he enters into dialogue with French authors, proving his continued relevance. At the same time that he attacks "dissection artists" ["Zergliederungs-Künstler"] (22), he also values their insights when he laments that typically only the hermaphrodite's external organs are dissected. Similarly, he both aligns with and distances himself from those who immerse themselves in books when he emphasizes his knowledge of the literature on hermaphrodites.

Burghart concludes his first-hand examination by saying that Drouart is a woman because of an imperforate penis and hidden vagina. He provides no illustration and argues that any new visual information would require Drouart "to die in Brieg to satisfy [his] curiosity and to dissect [him]" ["meinem Vorwitz zu Liebe zu Brieg sterben solten, damit ich sie möchte zergliedern können"] (23). Burghart notes that neither old nor new forms of inquiry lead to definitive pronouncements regarding sexually ambiguous humans.

Agency

Heinrich Friedrich Delius responded to Burghart in *Nachricht von dem besondern Hermaphroditen Drouart* [News of the special hermaphrodite Drouart], published in a 1765 collection of essays on natural sciences and pharmacy.[15] Delius engages Mertrud and Burghart and emphasizes that he is describing "what I myself observed" ["was ich selbst wahrgenommen habe"] (399). Unlike his predecessors, Delius presents Drouart not as a passive object but as a walking and talking human being. Delius describes how Drouart approached him during a lecture in Nürnberg:

> While I was occupied with the preparation of the inner female reproductive organs, the earlier mentioned Drouart arrived ... and offered ... to exhibit himself ... after I had examined him beforehand, I showed his relevant parts towards the end of my lecture.
> [Als ich aber mit der Zubereitung der weiblichen inneren Geburts Theile beschaeftigt war, meldete sich der erwehnte Drouart ... und erbot sich ... sich sehen zu lassen ... nachdem ich ihn vorher untersuchte, zeigte ich, zu Ende der Vorlesung, an demselben das gehörige.]
>
> (400)

When Delius describes Drouart's external genitals, he refers to them as "vagina," using Drouart's own words: "that he himself called 'vagine,' vagina, because this is what he had been told" ["den er selbst la vagine, die Scheide, weil man es ihm ohnehin so vorgesagt, nannte"] (402). The tension at the grammatical level—the reference to the female vagina and the use of a third-person male pronoun ("er") to refer to Drouart—positions Delius' text as a response to Burghart. In contrast to Burghart, who argued that Drouart was a woman, Delius conceives of him as a "deformed man" ["eine verstaltete Manns Person"] (404). Delius also enters into dialogue with Burghart's point that only a post-mortem autopsy would produce any new knowledge, when he reports that Drouart "laughed and said that if he died here, he would gladly give permission to be dissected" ["mit Lachen sagte, daß wann er hier stürbe, er es [anatomisieren] gern erlauben wollte"] (404). By emphasizing the limits of their knowledge, Burghart and Delius leave open the pathway for further inquiries and writings on Drouart.

Epistemological Aporia

The authors of the Drouart case studies created an increasingly dense textual web that could be rewritten endlessly. Vacherie's case study, for example, ends with "addenda," responding to his critics. He mentions that "a Negro Hermophradite [sic] from Guinea" (15) had served to invalidate the conclusion that Drouart was neither man nor woman.[16] Using the Guinean hermaphrodite as an analogy, Vacherie's critics argued that the opening to Drouart's vulva was in fact the urethra and that therefore Drouart was a man. Vacherie vehemently disagreed because "was this the Case, the Difference would be only local, and confined to those Parts of Generation" (17), yet the difference permeated Drouart's whole body. Vacherie searches for proof that hermaphrodites—humans with truly ambiguous genitalia—exist. In a footnote, he reports that "it is *pretended*, that at *Lyons, Rue Merciere*, there exists actually an Hermaphrodite truly perfect in both Sexes, but that by the Care of the Parents, who are wealthy merchants [this issue] ... must remain undecided" (14). Proof for the existence of true hermaphrodites remained elusive.

Drouart became a figure in other eighteenth-century writings on hermaphrodites, such as Antoine Ferrein's 1767 *Mémoire sur le véritable sexe de ceux qu'on appelle hermaphrodites* [Dissertation on the true sex of those that are called hermaphrodites], published in the *Mémoires de l'Académie Royale des Sciences*. Drouart serves to explain the case of a twelve-year-old child with ambiguous genitalia, "M.N." If found to be male, the child would become heir to a considerable fortune. Ferrein continues a line of reasoning opened by Vacherie's reference to a child of wealthy merchants. For Ferrein, the cases of the child and Drouart "shed light on each other" ["servent à s'éclaircir mutuellement"] (331). Ferrein examines Drouart in 1746, 1760, and 1761. A detailed (re)examination and comparison of both individuals and a survey of the relevant scholarship leads Ferrein to conclude that Drouart and "M.N." are both women: "one should not doubt ... that the internal parts and the uterus in particular, are the same in them as they are in other girls" ["on ne doit pas douter ... que les parties internes, & particulièrement la matrice, ne soient en eux comme chez les autres filles"] (337). In contrast to Vacherie, Ferrein concludes that no truly sexually ambiguous humans exist because careful inspection will allow for classification as male or female. Ferrein's title, which references "true sex" (330), is indicative of his belief in the power of the Enlightenment mind to solve the riddle of so-called hermaphrodites.

Drouart's story continued to be rewritten into the nineteenth century. As Drouart's body seems not to have been autopsied, his story remained open-ended. The public continued its voyeuristic interest in Drouart, while, for the medical community, Drouart's body also crystallized developments in the fields of anatomy, surgery, and obstetrics. The impossibility to decide on Drouart's sex was both the pre-condition for and the outcome of any scientific inquiry into his body. Drouart became the protagonist in a quasi-novelistic narrative that was disseminated widely in the medical marketplace of the eighteenth century. Like the novel, the genre of the case study allowed for the intense focus on one individual in unusual circumstances. It thereby mirrored the wider interest in determining an individual's place in the broader social, political, and economic order, which was undergoing significant changes over the course of the century.

Notes

1 "Hermaphrodite" refers to pre-twentieth-century representations of ambiguously sexed, or intersex, bodies.
2 See in particular Alice Dreger, Anne Fausto-Sterling, and Geertje Mak.
3 On the development of the market for popular scientific treatises, see Whitney Dirks-Schuster and George Rousseau.
4 This classificatory impulse can be contextualized with the gradual shift from the one- to the two-sex model described by Thomas Laqueur and Londa Schiebinger (*The Mind Has No Sex?*). According to the new logic of the two-sex model, the vagina became a mysterious organ requiring scrutiny and women needed to be controlled because their mysterious nature threatened the social order.
5 See Ruth Gilbert, Patrick Graille, and Maximilian Schochow for discussions of seventeenth- and eighteenth-century hermaphrodites.
6 Translations are mine, unless otherwise noted.
7 French allows male or female grammatical gender for "hermaphrodite."
8 See Hilger for a discussion of eighteenth-century authors' ambivalence towards the new demands for empirical science.
9 For an account of the pamphlet warfare between physicians and surgeons, see Gelfand 58–79.
10 See Courtney Thompson, Ruth Gilbert, Karen Harvey, and Valerie Traub.
11 Thomas Laqueur argues that Renaldo Columbus "discovered" the clitoris in 1559. See also Theresa Braunschneider, Felicity Nussbaum, Cath Sharrock, and Valerie Traub.
12 As Cathy McClive argues, erection and menstruation were thought to be possible in members of both sexes.
13 Bonner observes that there were significant differences in medical education in Britain, France, and Germany. Whereas in Britain and France, practical/clinical knowledge was gained outside the university, in Germany it was acquired within. French surgeons had a better reputation than German surgeons; they eventually created their own professional corporations. In Britain and France teaching medicine became a private enterprise. Generally, in France and Germany, the state had a bigger role in

medicine than in the Anglo-Saxon context, where private entrepreneurship was more pervasive. Despite these differences, however, the "sea change in attitudes toward practical training" (103) as well as the ensuing opportunities and anxieties permeated all contexts.

14 On this point, also see Roy Porter (293).
15 Delius' case study is included in *Fränkische Sammlungen von Anmerkungen aus der Naturlehre Arzneygelahrtheit Oekonomi und den damit verwandten Wissenschaften, einundvierzigtes Stück.*
16 See Hilger for a discussion of hermaphrodites in Britain's colonial territories.

Works Cited

Primary Texts

Burghart, D. Gottfried Heinrich. *Gründliche Nachricht an seinen Freund *** Von einem neuerlich gesehenen Hermaphroditen, Wobey zugleich etwas von der Medicinischen Mode erwähnet wird.* Breslau: Daniel Pietsch and Company, 1763.

Delius, Heinrich Friederich. "III. Nachricht von dem besondern Hermaphroditen Drouart." *Fränkische Sammlungen von Anmerkungen aus der Naturlehre Arzneygelahrtheit Oekonomi und den damit verwandten Wissenschaften, einundvierzigtes Stück.* Nuremberg: Bei George Peter Monat, 1765. 398–405.

Ferrein, Antoine. *Mémoire sur le véritable sexe de ceux qu'on appelle hermaphrodites. Mémoires de l'Académie Royale des Sciences.* Paris: Imprimerie Royale, 1767. 330–339.

Hoin, Jean Jacques Louis. *Nouvelle Description de l'Hermaphrodite Drouart, tel qu'on le voit à Dijon en août 1761.* Dijon: Veuve Coignard, 1761.

Mertrud, Antoine (and Jacques-Fabien Gautier d'Agoty). *Hermaphrodite, Dissertation au sujet de la fameuse hermaphrodite qui a paru aux yeux du public depuis environ trois mois, faite par le sieur Mertrud.* Paris: Berryer, 1749.

Morand, Sauveur-Francois. "Description d'un hermaphrodite, que l'on voyait à Paris en 1749." Jean-Michel Moreau, *Garçon et filles hermaphrodites vus et dessinés d'après nature par un des plus célèbres artistes et gravés avec tout le soin possible pour l'utilité des studieux.* Paris, 1773. (Reprint of the original published in *Mémoires de l'Académie Royale des Sciences de Paris,* 1750.)

Morand, Sauveur-Francois. *Discours dans lequel on prouve qu'il est nécessaire au chirurgien d'être lettré.* Paris, 1743.

Vacherie, M. *An Account of the Famous Hermaphrodite, or, Parisian Boy-Girl, Aged Sixteen, Named Michael-Anne Drouart.* London: Samuel Johnson, 1750.

Secondary Literature

Bonner, Thomas Neville. *Becoming a Physician: Medical Education in Britain, France, Germany, and the United States, 1750–1945.* New York: Oxford UP, 1995.

Braunschneider, Theresa. "The Macroclitoride, the Tribade and the Woman: Configuring Gender and Sexuality in English Anatomical Discourse." *Textual Practice* 13. 3 (1999): 509–532.

Dirks-Schuster, Whitney. "Print Culture and the Monstrous Hermaphrodite in Early Modern England." <www.inter-disciplinary.net/wp-content/uploads/2011/08/schus termpaper.pdf> Accessed 22 March 2015.

Dreger, Alice Domurat. *Hermaphrodites and the Medical Invention of Sex.* Cambridge: Harvard UP, 1998.

Fausto-Sterling, Anne. *Sexing the Body: Gender Politics and the Construction of Sexuality.* New York: Basic Books, 2000.

Gelfand, Toby. *Professionalizing Modern Medicine: Paris Surgeons and Medical Science and Institutions in the 18th Century.* London: Greenwood Press, 1980.

Geyer-Kordesch, Johanna. "German Medical Education in the Eighteenth Century: The Prussian Context and Its Influence." *William Hunter and the Eighteenth-Century Medical World.* Ed. W.F. Bynum and Roy Porter. Cambridge: Cambridge UP, 1985. 177–205.

Gilbert, Ruth. *Early Modern Hermaphrodites: Sex and Other Stories.* Houndmills: Palgrave Macmillan, 2002.

Graille, Patrick. *Les hermaphrodites au XVII et XVIIIième siècles.* Paris: Les Belles Lettres, 2001.

Harvey, Karen. *Reading Sex in the Eighteenth Century: Bodies and Gender in English Erotic Culture.* Cambridge: Cambridge UP, 2004.

Hilger, Stephanie. "Enlightenment Angst: James Parsons' *A Mechanical and Critical Enquiry into the Nature of Hermaphrodites* (1741)." *Taking Stock: Twenty-Five Years of Comparative Literary Research.* Ed. Norbert Bachleitner, Achim Hölter, and John McCarthy. Leiden: Brill, 2018. Forthcoming.

Laqueur, Thomas. *Making Sex: Body and Gender from the Greeks to Freud.* Cambridge: Harvard UP, 1990.

Mak, Geertje. *Doubting Sex: Inscriptions, Bodies, and Selves in Nineteenth-Century Hermaphrodite Case Histories.* Manchester: Manchester UP, 2012.

McClive, Cathy. *Menstruation and Procreation in Early Modern France.* London: Routledge, 2016.

Nussbaum, Felicity A. *Torrid Zones: Maternity, Sexuality, and Empire in Eighteenth-Century English Narratives.* Baltimore: Johns Hopkins UP, 1995.

Porter, Roy. *The Greatest Benefit to Mankind: A Medical History of Humanity.* New York: Norton, 1997.

Rousseau, George S. "Science Books and their Readers in the Eighteenth Century." *Books and their Readers in Eighteenth-Century England.* Ed. Isabel Rivers. New York: Leicester UP and St. Martin's P, 1982. 197–256.

Schiebinger, Londa. *The Mind Has No Sex? Women in the Origins of Modern Science.* Cambridge: Harvard UP, 1989.

Schiebinger, Londa. *Nature's Body: Gender in the Making of Modern Science.* New Brunswick: Rutgers UP, 2013.

Schochow, Maximilian. *Die Ordnung der Hermaphroditen-Geschlechter: Eine Genealogie des Geschlechtsbegriffs.* Berlin: Akademie Verlag, 2009.

Sharrock, Cath. "Hermaphroditism; or, 'the Erection of a New Doctrine': Theories of Female Sexuality in Eighteenth-Century England." *Paragraph* 17. 1 (1994): 38–48.

Spary, E.C. "Health and Medicine in the Enlightenment." *Oxford Handbook of the History of Medicine.* Ed. Mark Jackson. Oxford: Oxford UP, 2011. 82–99.

Thompson, Courtney E. "Questions of Genre: Picturing the Hermaphrodite in Eighteenth-Century France and England." *Eighteenth-Century Studies* 49. 3 (Spring 2016): 391–413.

Traub, Valerie. "The Psychomorphology of the Clitoris." *GLQ* 2(1995): 81–113.

4 Charting Intersex

Intersex Life-Writing and the Medical Record

Katelyn Dykstra

Intersex is a broad category that refers to an array of embodied traits that make it difficult to easily categorize bodies into social definitions of either male or female. Intersex may be located in the chromosomes, genitals, gonads, hormones, or secondary sex characteristics of the person so identified. In many parts of the world, intersex is designated a social emergency and physicians continue to recommend surgical or other medical solutions. Often parents are not given all the information they need to make an informed decision about their child's treatment because intersex is perceived by physicians as psychologically challenging. Therefore, secrets are also often kept from the intersex person. For all of these reasons, the Intersex Society of North America claims that "intersexuality is primarily a problem of shame and stigma, not of gender" (isna.org).[1] The "problem" is not indeterminate gender but the way our society, and by extension our medical establishment, shames and stigmatizes gender or sex non-conforming bodies.

We are entering an age in which intersex people are beginning to catalogue their catastrophic losses, personal and public struggles, and testimonies of thriving, in a public way. Their memoirs are being displayed on bookstore shelves, their narratives shared in heartfelt pleas for acceptance in YouTube videos, or on panels on the evening news about the continued use of cosmetic genital surgeries on children too young to consent. While sociologists briefly reference these memoirs in their studies of the biomedicalization of intersex bodies,[2] there are few in-depth studies of the texts themselves because literary scholars do not consider them as worthy of serious study. That intersex memoirs have, for the most part, not been examined in meaningful ways in literary studies[3] speaks to both the invisibility of intersex in our society and the generic instability of the genre of the memoir, situated on the border between history and literature. This chapter, by using the tools of close textual analysis, considers not *what* is lost for intersex people but "*how* that loss is apprehended" (Eng and Kazanjian 6, emphasis in original) and explores the methods used by intersex writers to convey their traumas.

This chapter engages the preexisting work on autobiographical trauma writing done by Leigh Gilmore, who, drawing on the insights of John Paul Eakin, Sidonie Smith, and Julia Watson, asks how writing about one's trauma can be taken seriously as "truth" at the same time that it is haunted by the effects of trauma that often shatter the psyche. As Dina Georgis writes of trauma writing, "trauma is most certainly a crisis of knowledge. Language fails. As such, the past is reconstructed between what we know and remember and what is lost to memory" (10). The writer's process of bringing these fragmented traumas to the page affects the reader, often politically. Psychoanalysis therefore, through its attention to both conscious and unconscious construction of memory, provides a productive tool for examining the trauma of medicalization experienced by intersex writers.

An example of intersex trauma writing can be found in the 2015 issue of the journal *Narrative Inquiry in Bioethics*. In this special issue on intersex, Georgiann Davis, a prominent intersex scholar and sociologist, collected and published a "Narrative Symposium," to which I will refer as *The Symposium* hereafter. *The Symposium* consists of the brief (two to three page) personal stories of thirteen people with intersex traits from disparate "race/ethnicity, age, gender identity, nationality, religious observance, diagnosis, and treatment" backgrounds, in an effort to "normalize, in a positive sense, [intersex] experiences" ("Narrative Symposium" 89). As Davis points out, this narrative intervention is important because people with intersex traits have "historically been the objects, rather than the producers, of knowledge about [intersex] bodies and experiences" (89). I will focus on three of these narratives: Lynnell Stephani Long's "Still I Rise," Pidgeon Pagonis's "The Son They Never Had," and Karen A. Walsh's "'Normalizing' Intersex Didn't Feel Normal or Honest to Me." I chose these particular texts because of the similarities in the ways they negotiate their relationships to their medical care team, their memories, and their commitment to activism and community resulting from the surgical alteration of their bodies.

These texts constitute an important contribution to the small genre of inter-sex life-writing, which has featured mainly writers that have not been subject to normalizing genital surgeries such as Thea Hillman's *Intersex (For Lack of a Better Word)* (2008) and Hida Viloria's *Born Both: An Intersex Life* (2017). The voices in *The Symposium* are therefore important because they provide insight into the process of medicalization and its effects from a first-person perspective that includes voices of people of color such as Pagonis and Long. In these memoirs, the material object of the medical chart figures prominently. The reappearance of the chart in these texts does not function as an empty signifier, but as an object with its own "vitalism," as Jane Bennett would have it in her discussion of what she calls "vibrant objects," "entities not entirely reducible to the contexts in which (human) subjects set them, never entirely exhausted by their semiotics" (5). Attending to objects *as* objects in texts allows us to see the way they act on humans in a way we would not be able to otherwise. For example, the focus on the medical chart records the significance not just of the words written in the chart but the import of the way the chart-object moves from the space of the physician's office, which constantly subjects the intersex body to medical scrutiny, to the private space of the intersex patient. In addition, for the author of the memoir, the acquisition of the medical chart allows for a move from individual melancholia to collective, militant mourning and is therefore central to the creation of a politicized intersex community. In "Mourning and Melancholia," Sigmund Freud presents mourning as the normal response to the loss of a "loved person, or the loss of some abstraction which has taken the place of one, such as one's country, liberty, ideal, and so on" (243). While mourning may make us strange for the moment, eventually reality takes over, and we are able to get back to the business of living our normal lives. The pathological response, in contrast, is melancholia, a troubled, ceaseless mourning for the lost object or objects.[4]

Melancholia as it exists in early Freud is useful as an analytical concept for the intersex experience. Growing up with so much secrecy surrounding their bodies, with scars without any explanation, with repeated exposure to the medical gaze, the intersex person bears a sense of loss, but without the words to name it, and therefore without any method to process it. The lost object—the non-injured body, the "whole" body, which can also be read as the "disparaged object" of normal heteronormative masculinity (Eng 1277) which the intersex body, because of its sexed difference, cannot perform—is incorporated into the ego. But once the intersex person is able to access the object of their medical chart, they can name themselves as intersex and move out of this particular early-Freudian sense of melancholia and into what Douglas Crimp describes as a militant state of mourning. Crimp's formulation of "mourning and militancy" (137) sheds light on a particular kind of collective mourning that occurs in a moment of political and social crisis, to understand the importance of the physical handling of the chart for the intersex author's move from individual melancholia to what Eng refers to as a collective "mourning without end" (Eng and Han 670). Crimp describes how, in the face of AIDS, some gay men slid into a moralistic melancholia, where the loss of loved ones was too much to bear, and so the melancholic person rejected the *jouissance*[5] of gay life which they associated with the disease. Crimp, however, advocates for a militant mourning that champions "queer responsibility" which enthusiastically endorses riotous sex in the face of the disease.[6] The concept of "queer responsibility" is useful for intersex because those who claim their chart and who write their story do so out of a newfound love of their bodies, a "queer responsibility," which aims to spread the love of their identities as intersex and to practice a radical politics of care for their own bodies and for those of others.

In their brief, autobiographical account of their life, entitled "The Son They Never Had," Pidgeon Pagonis describes their first meeting with intersex activist Lynnell Stephani Long: "Go ahead, say 'I'm intersex,'" Long encourages Pagonis. After some hesitation, Pidgeon mumbles "'I'm intersex.'" "'What? I can't hear you,' Lynnell said with a smile. 'I'm INTERSEX.' 'There you go. Next step is to get your records'" ("Narrative Symposium" 105).[7] As this example shows, the medical chart is an object which is physically taken, hidden, and recovered as part of a liberatory process of constructing the self apart from the medical industrial complex.[8] The medical record provides the intersex writer with a diagnosis, which in turn establishes an identity as intersex and allows for the disentangling of their body from the medical establishment. Moreover, as part of this process of learning about themselves, often the chart provides concrete proof of physical and psychological wounding that may or may not be remembered by the intersex person. For the traumatized intersex person, the act of writing becomes an act of rewriting, either of their personal history or of the medical history, which is riddled with gaps.

Gaps are representative of both lost memory, and the lost object that holds the memory—the medical chart. Thus, when the chart is found, read, and its contents internalized by the intersex patient reader, a move out of Freud's early formulation of melancholia is possible. Accessing the chart and reading it, which may give the intersex person a name for their bodies and a disclosure of the medical procedures that were performed on their bodies without their full knowledge or consent, allows the writer to imagine and, in some cases, experience a community of intersex people, as the HIV diagnosis was able to do for Douglas Crimp. However, the chart then also presents a double bind where the author has to repeat medical terminology for their body in the form of the word "intersex" to find a community that allows for the onset of collective mourning.

For some of the writers in *The Symposium*, accessing their chart is difficult. Because many of them feel that the truth hidden in the chart is vital to their formation as a subject, this act of withholding is damaging. In her short memoir for *The Symposium*, "'Normalizing' Intersex Didn't Feel Normal or Honest to Me," Karen A. Walsh writes that "truthful disclosure didn't come to me about my biology and what was done to me as an infant until I was 33, when I forced the issue by removing my medical records from my endocrinologist's office" ("Narrative Symposium" 119). Walsh had found references to herself in a medical journal published in 1960, wherein the doctor describes her anatomy as an infant and the procedure he performed on her, but gives no information about either the reasons for performing the surgery or its impact. The only reason that the doctor provided was that Walsh's gonads could become malignant, but more importantly that there was concern about Walsh following a "'normal psychosexual pattern'" (120). The goal for Walsh's physician was "normal psychic development" (120), which, however, as Walsh points out, never occurred. Instead, Walsh experiences extreme disassociation because of her inability to remember important events in her life as a result of her traumatic surgical experiences and more importantly the lies her physicians and her family told her at the request of those physicians. About her large abdominal scars, she writes:

> Growing up, I was treated like a fascinoma and a lab rat at a major teaching hospital on the East Coast. All I learned from those doctors as a young kid was what it feels like to be ogled, photographed, and probed by a roomful of white-coated male doctors. Disassociation made itself my friend, and helped me cope through annual genital and anal exams and probing. I thought I was a freak and I felt completely powerless to protect myself from them and their "care."
>
> (120)

A key component to Freud's theory of melancholia in "Mourning and Melancholia," is an "extraordinary diminution in [the individual's] self-regard, an impoverishment of his ego on a grand scale." Freud observes that the "patient represents his ego to us as worthless, incapable of any achievement and morally despicable; he reproaches himself, vilifies himself and expects to be cast out and punished" (246). The unexplained loss of power has left Walsh in a state of melancholy. She feels like a "freak" and takes a moralistic stand against herself in a process of dis-association. She also thinks that she is responsible for protecting herself from her physicians, and her inability to do so perpetuates her sense that her ego is "incapable of achievement" (246). She therefore allows herself to continue to be "punished" into gender conformity by physicians through their repeated acts of "care."

Later in life, Walsh is hospitalized after her vagina rips during intercourse. She writes that had she known the hidden information about her genital anatomy, she would have been more cautious.[9] Following this literal tearing of her body, Walsh is compelled to act. Walsh explains how she removed the medical records from her endocrinologist's office after he "stonewalled" (120) her, refusing to tell her the truth about her intersex trait and how it had been medicalized. She refuses to accept this rebuke, and in response removes her medical chart from his office and reads it in the parking lot (122). This act transforms her intersexuality from a pathology projected onto her body by the medical establishment to an element of her identity that she owns. By removing the chart and taking it with her into her own private space, she is also *de facto* moving her body from object of medical management to liberated subject in charge of her own destiny. She has reclaimed medical language for herself.

The medical chart, or record, lays bare the evidence of wounding. It makes plain all that has been done to the intersex person. Pidgeon Pagonis's piece, "The Son They Never Had," includes selections of their medical records. These records appear before Pagonis discusses their knowledge of being intersex. They foreshadow the pain to come. The first record reads:

> Medical Record 6/6/86—Informant: Mother and grandmother Immediate Complaint: Abnormal genitals Present Illness: Jennifer has been considered to be entirely well until exam last week by pediatrician who noted enlarged clitoris and small vaginal opening. Female Genitalia: Clitoral enlargement of 1.5 cm. Sex assignment as a female is entirely appropriate.
>
> ("Narrative Symposium" 103)

In the brief scene recounted earlier, Pagonis meets Lynnell Stephani Long, who tells them to say they are intersex. Once they do, Long explains that "the next step is for you to get your records" (105). By including bits of these records for the reader to see, Pagonis gives us a snippet of the physician's diagnostic thought process. Pagonis makes it clear that their body was "considered to be entirely well until" it was not. That is, until an "enlarged clitoris and small vaginal opening are found." This discovery, for the medical establishment, means that the body is unwell, and is now open to medicalization.

What is unique about Pagonis's piece is that we see them respond to their own medical chart directly by including excerpts from it. They explain how each procedure felt before and after it happened, which renders visible what is typically deleted from the medical record—the patient's feelings. For example, the surgery Pagonis undergoes at the age of eleven to "correct Jennifer's [Pagonis's prior first name] problem with urination" becomes an extremely traumatic moment for them. The chart continues: "At the same time, [Dr. F] is considering doing a vaginoplasty" (103). It is Dr. F who is considering vagino- plasty, not Pagonis or her family. Pagonis describes the preparations for surgery:

> I was being prepared for anesthesia. The doctors came into the room to tell me what was going to happen next. "We noticed that your vagina is smaller than other girls'. While we're in the operating room fixing your urethra, we can also make a small incision in your vagina to make it larger. This way, you'll be able to have sex with your husband when you're older. Does that sound good?"[10]

Pagonis writes that, in response, they let out a "shameful 'yes.'" When they wake up from surgery, they write that they were "no longer a child" (104).

By relating their own experience as well as the physician's justification of the procedures, Pagonis allows us to see how the chart fills in gaps in their own story. As a young child, they did not understand what was happening to them or why. But in retrospect, writing their story alongside the medical chart enables them to link "Dr. F is considering a vaginoplasty" to the hetero- normative imperative to "have sex with [their] husband." By understanding the physicians' impetus to alter her body to make it more (hetero)normative Pago- nis is able to construct a legible trajectory of their own life. Moreover, they emerge as activists, as manifested in publishing their life story in *The Symposium*, to stop the same practices being enacted on others.

To construct a legible life-narrative is, in many ways, the goal of psychoanalysis. Because of the lack of information given to the intersex person their attachments are melancholic prior to the discovery of their medical record. There is no place to ground the pain because there are no memories. Arthur Frank reads this shift in understanding one's experience after reading the medical record as an editorial shift in one's narrative. He claims they now have a "new story" which is not more or less "true" than the old one, but fills in blank spaces when a person may have been sedated or anesthetized during surgery or may simply not have been told the whole story (23). An extension of this feeling of knowing what really happened is the relief of having a diagnosis, a legitimate way to explain, or address, their body and what has happened to it. Often the reading of the chart marks a distinct shift from helplessness to agency. The path from melancholia to collective mourning, then, is one from a state in which the loss of power is unexplained and leaves the subject helpless, to one in which the loss of power is understood and can be mourned.

Lynnell Stephani Long, who mentored Pagonis in their struggle to find, process, and write about their medical records, writes about her own difficulties trying to find her medical records in her text "Still I Rise." But first, she writes: "It wasn't until I got sick in 1995, however, that I found out that there was a medical term to describe me. I was intersex" ("Narrative Symposium" 101). She explains how she began to understand her identity:

> I started researching my medical history in 1996 and after buying a computer I began to search the internet. It wasn't until I saw Cheryl Chase (aka Bo Laurant) on television that I had a name for what was "wrong" with me. I am intersex.
>
> (102)

Her research acts as a conduit, like the medical chart, to identity formation. Before naming herself as intersex she did not know what she was. Long explains that during childhood she thought she was a girl until her mother "beat it out of me. Literally" (101). Lynnell is subjected to multiple treatments that are not fully explained to her, and that she cannot explain to her friends. The physicians never ask her what she wants, but they continue to work to make her into a legible boy (101). This secrecy, compounded by the work of the physicians to make her into a boy, leads Lynnell to abuse drugs and to attempt suicide.

The act of researching her own medical history, by which she is able to access a "diagnosis" as intersex, encapsulates the process during which the individual trauma of secrecy and shame moves into a collective sense of mourning. Long is able to find others like her, such as Cheryl Chase. Thus, constructing a community of people, if only online, through which to process her sense of loss—loss of agency, loss of a childhood in the "wrong" gender, the loss of body parts, the sense of loss at not having a mother that confirmed and supported her gender identity. Moreover, through the process of writing in *The Symposium*, Long is participating in Crimp's notion of "queer responsibility" whereby she is not allowing the shame of her diagnosis to maintain a melancholic attachment to her losses, but instead begins to mourn them.

It is tempting to refer to this sustained militant mourning as melancholic because of its inability to successfully overcome the loss. Yet Long's example shows the intertwining of melancholia's persistence along with collective mourning's move away from individual self-harm and suicidation and into activism and advocacy within a community of other mourners. Walsh, Pagonis, and Long move out into the world with renewed vigor to address the harm done to them and advocate for others. In brief, these writers' ability to claim the term "intersex" for themselves, and therefore to move out of melancholia and into a militant state of collective mourning by accessing their medical record, places their texts under the heading of "intersex" writing. Their goal is the cessation of unnecessary medical management of future and present intersex bodies. Butler writes that loss is necessary for the formulation of marginalized communities because it is that very sense of loss and trauma that creates the community. The losses sustained at the hands of medical professionals compel intersex authors to write, and, through the narration of their losses, a genre of intersex life-writing emerges.

Notes

1 ISNA was disbanded in 2008 in an effort to turn away from the term "intersex" in favor of DSDs (Disorders of Sexual Development). The organizers at ISNA posted on their website that they were starting a new organization, the Accord Alliance, which marked a moving away from ISNA's "scrappy" and "controversial" roots in activism and towards a more collaborative approach with the medical industrial complex in an effort to more successfully argue for intersex people within medical spaces. However, the switch from "intersex" to "DSD"s has had a tremendous impact on the intersex activist community. Some activists feel that DSD's reliance on the word "disorder" further pathologizes intersex bodies; as a result they have formed new organizations, including OII (Organization Intersex International) which maintains the "scrappy" and "confrontational" origins of ISNA and continues its disruption of stark gender and sex categories. I align my own work with the aims of OII and reject the notion that intersex bodies are pathological. I therefore use the term "intersex" exclusively.

2 While there is a distinct absence of work in literary studies on intersex, there is a growing number of texts that use intersex stories in sociological studies of the bio-medicalization of intersex bodies. Most notable among these studies are Susanne Kessler's *Lessons Learned from the Intersexed*; Sharon Preves's *Intersex and Identity: The Contested Self*; Anne Fausto-Sterling's *Sexing the Body: Gender Politics and the Construction of Sexuality*; Katrina Karkazis' *Fixing Sex: Intersex, Medical Authority, and Lived Experience*; Georgiann Davis' *Contesting Intersex: The Dubious Diagnosis*; and Ellen K. Feder's *Making Sense of Intersex: Changing Ethical Perspectives in Biomedicine*. Morgan Holmes has also published two foundational texts on intersex, each with a more interdisciplinary approach, *Intersex: A Perilous Difference* and *Critical Intersex*, along with numerous articles. Historical considerations of intersex include Elizabeth Reis's *Bodies in Doubt: An American History of Intersex* and Alice Dreger's *Hermaphrodites and the Medical Invention of Sex*.

3 Two texts have recently been published out of North American Studies programs in Germany. The first is Viola Amato's *Intersex Narratives: Shifts in the Representation of Intersex Lives in North American Literature and Popular Culture* (2016). The second is Michaela Koch's *Discursive Intersexions: Myth, Medicine, and Memoir* (2017).

4 David Eng has uncovered a later discussion of melancholia in Freud in which he is unable to maintain the distinction between pathological mourning (melancholia) and healthy mourning. In *The Ego and the Id*, Eng reminds us, Freud revises his position on melancholia and comes to understanding melancholia as necessary to the formation of the ego. "As such," Eng writes, "there can be no ego without, or prior to, melancholia" (1277). It is, therefore, possible to understand that melancholia is normative, "as a constitutive psychic mechanism engendering subjectivity itself" (1277). Eng's re-examination of these categories makes evident that mourning and melancholia are not binary opposites on the poles of a normal or pathological response to trauma and loss. Instead, they intertwine. However, Freud's early formulation of melancholia allows me to highlight the distinct move away from individual suffering and toward a collective and militant method of narrating loss. It is my contention that the move away from individual melancholia is what allows for intersex trauma writing because it makes space for the writer to enter a genre of politicized intersex life-writing.

5 Crimp uses *jouissance* here in the Lacanian sense. Lacan defines *jouissance* as not necessarily the satisfaction of a need or a desire, but the satisfaction of a drive. The drive, according to Lacan, is "something extremely complex" that "can't be reduced to the complexity of the instinct" but, instead, it is a kind of "energy" (Lacan in Braunstein 104).

6 Iain Morland takes issue with the focus on pleasure in queer theory, as exemplified by Douglas Crimp. He argues that such a focus sidesteps the post-surgical, potential atypically sensate intersex body. My use of Crimp in the context of intersex life writing allows me to move his focus on pleasurable sex to the pleasure of self-love as an act of political opposition to genital surgeries, specifically by those too young to consent.

7 I adhere to Pagonis's plural pronouns.

8 Most intersex people are not given access to their medical charts until later in life. Some need legal action or the threat of legal action to get access (Blair 89; Truffer 111), while others have resorted to taking them from a doctor's office (Walsh, "Narrative Symposium" 121).

9 Psychoanalyst Myra Hird cites a study that argued that telling subjects that they were intersex was less psychologically damaging than withholding that information (1080).

10 The moments of divergence between the physician's justification and Pagonis's own experience expose the power imbalance between them.

Works Cited

Amato, Viola. *Intersex Narratives: Shifts in the Representation of Intersex Lives in North American Literature and Popular Culture.* Bielefeld: Transcript Verlag, 2016.

Bennett, Jane. *Vibrant Matter: A Political Ecology of Things.* Durham: Duke UP, 2010.

Blair, Konrad. "When Doctors Got it Wrong." *Narrative Inquiry in Bioethics* 5. 2 (2015): 89–92.

Braunstein, Néstor A. "Desire and Jouissance in the Teaching of Lacan." *The Cambridge Companion to Lacan.* Ed. Jean-Michel Rabaté. Cambridge: Cambridge UP, 2003. 102–112.

Butler, Judith. "Afterword: After Loss, What Then?" *Loss: The Politics of Mourning.* Ed. David Eng and David Kazanjian. Los Angeles: U of California P, 2003. 467–473.

Crimp, Douglas. *Melancholia and Moralism: Essays on AIDS and Queer Politics.* Cambridge: MIT P, 2002.

Davis, Georgiann. *Contesting Intersex: The Dubious Diagnosis.* New York: New York UP, 2015.

Davis, Georgiann, ed. "Narrative Symposium." Special issue of *Narrative Inquiry in Bioethics* 5. 2(2015).

Dreger, Alice. *Hermaphrodites and the Medical Invention of Sex.* Boston: Harvard UP, 2000.

Dreger, Alice Domurat. *Intersex in the Age of Ethics.* Hagerstown: Univ Pub Group, 1999.

Eng, David L. "Melancholia in the Late 20th Century." *Signs* 25. 4(Summer 2000): 1275–1281.

Eng, David and Shinhee Han. "A Dialogue on Racial Melancholia." *Psychoanalytic Dialogues* 10. 4(2000): 667–700.

Eng, David and David Kazanjian. "Introduction: Mourning Remains." *Loss: The Politics of Mourning.* Los Angeles: U of California P, 2003. 1–25.

Fausto-Sterling, Anne. *Sexing the Body: Gender Politics and the Construction of Sexuality.* New York: Basic Books, 2000.

Feder, Ellen K. *Making Sense of Intersex: Changing Ethical Perspectives in Biomedicine.* Bloomington: Indiana UP, 2014.

Frank, Arthur. *The Wounded Storyteller: Body, Illness, Ethics.* Chicago: U of Chicago P, 2013.

Freud, Sigmund. "Mourning and Melancholia." *Standard Edition of the Complete Psychological Works of Sigmund Freud.* Vol. XIV. London: Hogarth, 1948. 243–258.

Georgis, Dina. *The Better Story: Queer Affects from the Middle East.* New York: SUNY P, 2014.

Gilmore, Leigh. *The Limits of Autobiography: Trauma and Testimony.* Ithaca: Cornell UP, 2001.

Hillman, Thea. *Intersex (For Lack of a Better Word).* San Francisco: Manic D Press, 2008.

Hird, Myra J. "Considerations for a Psychoanalytic Theory of Gender Identity and Sexual Desire: The Case of Intersex." *Signs* 28. 4 (Summer 2003): 1067–1092.

Holmes, Morgan M., ed. *Critical Intersex.* London: Routledge, 2009.

Holmes, Morgan. *Intersex: A Perilous Difference.* Cranbury: Rosemont, 2008.

Karkazis, Katrina. *Fixing Sex: Intersex, Medical Authority, and Lived Experience.* Durham: Duke UP, 2008.

Kessler, Suzanne. *Lessons from the Intersexed.* New Brunswick: Rutgers UP, 1998.

Koch, Michaela. *Discursive Intersexions: Myth, Medicine, and Memoir.* Bielefeld: Transcript Verlag, 2017.

Morland, Iain. "What Can Queer Theory Do for Intersex?" *GLQ* 15. 2(2009): 285–312.

Preves, Sharon E. *Intersex and Identity: The Contested Self.* New Brunswick: Rutgers UP, 2003.

Reis, Elizabeth. *Bodies in Doubt: An American History of Intersex.* Baltimore: Johns Hopkins UP, 2009.

Truffer, Daniela. "It's a Human Rights Issue!" *Narrative Inquiry in Bioethics 5.* 2(2015): 111–114.

Viloria, Hida. *Born Both: An Intersex Life.* Abingdon: Hachette Books, 2017.

5   Narrating Sex Change in Iran

Transsexuality and the Politics of Documentary Film

Najmeh Moradiyan-Rizi

Introduction

In Western imagery, Iran has been predominantly registered as an exotic Oriental country with an ancient civilization and a traditional culture rooted in religion. This exoticizing and Orientalizing approach is vivid in numerous Western travelogues, paintings, and photographs of the nineteenth and early twentieth centuries, and later, in documentary films, television news productions, and journalistic reports. In regard to the historical interconnectedness of photography, Orientalism, and Western—mostly European—imperial projects in the Middle East, Ali Behdad asserts:

> Although photography of "the Orient" was indebted to the earlier literary and painterly representations of the region and was deeply invested in the discourse of exoticism, the indexical quality of these photographs made them factual and truthful representations in the minds of European audiences, who voraciously consumed them.
>
> (1–2)

The photographic images of the Middle East were not only used to render the Orient transparent and accessible, but they "were [also] inscribed in an ethnological system of differentiation and classification that made them both legible and desirable as images of cultural alterity" (Behdad 5). Since the invention of the cinematic medium, Western-produced documentary films and news footage have assumed the role previously played by photographs: they manipulate the notion of objective and truthful representation to perpetuate a mode of ethnic hierarchy that reinforces Western supremacy over the people and cultures of the Middle East. In regard to Iran, Hamid Naficy divides Western—mainly British and American—filmic approaches to pre-Revolutionary Iran into two major categories, "Exotic Underdeveloped (1900–1941)" and "Strategic Modern (1942–1979)" (218). Naficy argues that these films "have tended both to emphasize the supremacy of West over the ancient, backward East and to support the evolving policies and ideologies toward Iran held by the Western governments and their multi-national corporations" (217).[1]

Since the 1979 Islamic Revolution Western media representations have adopted a reductive discourse depicting Iran as a conservative, Islamic country rather than presenting its complex social, political, religious, and cultural contexts. I consider these portrayals neo-Orientalist visual tropes of stereotyping. Neo-Orientalism, as described by Ali Behdad and Juliet Williams, projects:

> a mode of representation that, while indebted to classical Orientalism, engenders new tropes of othering. ... [N]eo-Orientalism entails a popular mode of representing, a kind of *doxa* about the Middle East and Muslims that is disseminated, thanks to new technologies of communication, throughout the world.
>
> (284)[2]

Even documentaries that claim to show a more nuanced glimpse of Iran, such as Lisa Truitt's *Iran: Behind the Veil* (1999) or Nahid Persson Sarvestani's *Prostitution Behind the Veil* (2004), use Orientalist titles that reify a hegemonic Western perspective and emphasize traditional themes like gender repression.[3] The rise of Western media's attention to post-Revolutionary Iran, therefore, has left little room for the nuanced discussion of women's, gay, lesbian, queer, and transsexual lives beyond a focus on the violation of their rights. By analyzing aesthetic and discursive tropes of a Western-produced documentary film, *Be Like Others* (2008), directed by Iranian-American filmmaker Tanaz Eshaghian, I focus on the issue of transsexuality in Iran in order to show how neo-Orientalist ideology and rhetoric do not allow for a nuanced documentary representation of Iranian transsexuals. This chapter thus challenges the film's reductive approach to transsexuality in Iran, which aligns it with homosexuality, and highlights instead the complexities and particularities of sex change in the country as a way to provide an understanding of transsexual specificities pertinent to Iran's socio-cultural context. In doing so, the chapter addresses three major issues. First, it highlights the socio-cultural and religious specificities of Iranian society in relation to the implementation of the Islamic Shi'i laws after the 1979 Islamic Revolution and emphasizes the nuances of gender relations and subjectivities, particularly in regard to transsexuals, to challenge the reductive Western discourses of gender repression and victimhood. Second, it questions the heteronormative approach of the Iranian state to gender identification, which treats transsexuality as illness and transsexuals as patients. And finally, it foregrounds the complexity of the formation of transsexual identity in post-Revolutionary Iran, where gender, sexual, and cultural norms are constantly being negotiated and/or contested.

Western media is attracted to the issue of transsexuality in Iran mainly because of the assumption that Iran "is a place of sex and gender repression and regression" (Bucar and Enke 309), where human rights in general and women's, gay, lesbian, queer, and transsexual rights in particular are often violated. The Islamic Republic of Iran has offered a religiously and legally sanctioned approach, which considers transsexuals as patients suffering from a gender abnormality that can be cured by psychotherapy, hormone therapy, and sex reassignment surgery (SRS). Both Western and official Iranian discourses ignore Iranian transsexuals' subjectivity in defining their own sexual, gender, and social identity. As Afsaneh Najmabadi points out:

> Conservative forces in both Iran and the West have a common stake in ignoring the lively reform discourse and history of progressive activism within contemporary Iran that offers alternative notions of rights within an Islamic society and of alternative modes of living a Muslim life.
>
> ("Transing and Transpassing" 25)

While "[s]urgeries to alter congenital intersex conditions were reported in the Iranian press as early as 1930" (Najmabadi, "Transing and Transpassing" 25), domestic and international media and documentary coverage of transsexual discourses and representations in Iran have dramatically increased since the 2000s. Documentary films such as Mitra Farahani's *Just a Woman* (*Juste une femme*, 2002), Zohreh Shayesteh's *Inside Out* (2006), Elhum Shakerifar's *Roya and Omid* (2008), and Tanaz Eshaghian's *Be Like Others* (2008) document the experiences of Iranian transsexuals. Journalistic reports describe Iran as one of the sex-change capitals of the world. "Iran carries out more gender reassignment operations than any other country in the world besides Thailand," writes Dan Littauer (*Gay Star News*). Mainstream Western media reports including the BBC's "The Gay People Pushed to Change Their Gender," *The Guardian*'s "Iran's Persecution of Gay Community Revealed," and *The Huffington Post*'s "Iran's Sex Change Operations Provided Nearly Free-Of-Cost" underestimate the religiously and legally sanctioned role of sex reassignment surgery in Iran by highlighting the banishment of homosexuality derived from the Islamic interpretations.[4] Thus these mainstream media reports omit the complexities of Iranian society and its Islamic Shi'i laws, which paradoxically reside at the heart of their arguments. In the same vein, the internationally acclaimed documentary *Be Like Others* (2008) attempts to tackle the seemingly contradictory role of transsexuality and SRS in Iran in the context of the crackdown on homosexuality. Yet, as I argue, the reading of transsexuality in Iran within a homosexual context is problematic as it ignores the complexity of social, cultural, and religious structures in Iran, and excludes transsexual subjectivity and identity, thus reinforcing a heterosexual/homosexual binary. By distinguishing the body narratives of Iranian transsexuals in three distinct spaces presented in the film—society, family, and the clinic—I show how the transsexual body subverts Iran's gender-segregated social boundaries, heteronormative and hierarchical family structures, and the medical rhetoric of disorderliness and illness that seeks to cure transsexual persons. In contrast to the official Iranian rhetoric of abnormality and the Western narrative of oppression, which define the transsexual body as a passive object of technology, medicine, and society, I provide a counter-narrative that points to the recognition of transsexual subjectivity and identity in Iranian society.

Transsexuality or Homosexuality: A Counter-Narrative

Transgender studies often seeks to correct the reading of transsexuality within a homosexual context in order to fill the discursive gaps and ruptures of gay/lesbian studies and feminist studies. Elhum Shakerifar argues that "the frequent amalgamation of sexual orientations and gender attributes under the banner of Lesbian Gay Bisexual and Transgender (LGBT) communities" conflates different, yet related, issues of sexual desire—in the case of gay, lesbian, and bisexual—and sexual embodiment—in the case of transsexuals—and risks the isolation of transsexual subjectivity in visual and discursive contexts (329). Similar to the fact that feminist scholars came to see the category of "women" as "too much a universalization of white, Western, straight women" (Scott 22), which overlooks women's differences in various geo-cultural contexts, and hints at a confirmation of binary of sexes (male/female) and sexual difference, the readings of transsexuality in relation to gay and lesbian identity "reify the heterosexual/homosexual binary" (Nagel 116). Similarly, Judith Butler challenges the equation of homosexuality and transsexuality/transgenderism by asserting that "cross-gendered identification is not the exemplary paradigm for thinking about homosexuality, although it may be one" ("Critically Queer" 25).

In *Second Skins: The Body Narratives of Transsexuality* Jay Prosser observes, "Transsexuality consists in entering into a lengthy, formalized, and normally substantive transition: a correlated set of corporeal, psychic, and social changes" (4). This transition problematizes both the constructed discourse and the stereotypical visual representation of sex, gender, and sexuality in relation to transsexual embodiment, which are presented in *Be Like Others*. The film starts with three consecutive white titles, written on a black screen, which set the filmic narrative and approach throughout the documentary (emphasis mine):

> - In the Islamic Republic of Iran, a country with *strict* social mores and *traditional* values, sex change operations are legal.
> - Ayatollah Khomeini issued a *religious* edict over 20 years ago decreeing sex change operations are allowed for diagnosed transsexuals.
> - *Homosexuality* is punishable by death.

The titles lead to some long shots of Tehran before the camera enters the Mirdamad Surgical Center, where most sex reassignment surgeries in Iran occur. In regard to the documentary genre's perspective Bill Nichols writes:

> [D]ocumentaries may represent the world in the same way a lawyer may represent a client's interests: they put the case for a particular view or interpretation of evidence before us. In this sense documentaries do not simply stand for others, representing them in ways they could not do themselves, but rather they more actively make a case or argument.
>
> (*Introduction* 4)

The titles in *Be Like Others*, thus, actively highlight the unlikeliness of SRS in Iran, a country with traditional and strict social values, and present a reading of transsexuality in relation to homosexuality. Further, the titles juxtapose the legal and religiously sanctioned process of SRS with the banishment of homosexuality in Iran, arguing that the acceptability of SRS in Iran is an attempt at regulating homosexuality.

Sex reassignment surgery was first religiously sanctioned by the Arabic *fatwa* of Ayatollah Khomeini in the 1960s while he was in political exile during the Pahlavi regime. After the 1979 Islamic Revolution, Khomeini, the founder of the Islamic Republic, re-issued his *fatwa* in Persian and "set in motion the process that culminated in new state-sanctioned medicolegal procedures regarding transsexuality" (Najmabadi, "Transing and Transpassing" 26). Thus, legal, medical, and public sectors in Iran essentially derive their approach to the acceptability of transsexuality and SRS from this religious edict.[5] In fact, for some Shi'i scholars the religious sanctioning of SRS finds its root in the notion of soul/body distinction, which can be read as "gender identity/sex" distinction. In this context, a transsexual is considered a patient whose soul is trapped in the wrong body, and therefore, has the right to surgery in order to match his/her soul and body moving toward a "perfected," "normal" personhood. In *Be Like Others*, the cleric Kariminiya, a theological expert on transsexuality, considers SRS an alignment with nature's order, stating:

> If changing your gender was to be considered a sin because you are changing God's natural order, then all of our daily tasks would be sins! You take wheat and turn it into flour and turn that into bread. ... Why is that not considered a sin?

This ideological point of view therefore supports transsexuals to adapt one of the male/female sexual categories in accordance with their gender identity. However, SRS is not synonymous with "realness," because the post-op transsexual body is a mere fabrication of sexual difference. In this regard, Prosser writes, "Because sex has become irreducible not only to the sex organs accessible to surgical remolding but to the body itself, the transsexual's attempted sex reassignment may serve to illustrate the very failure of sexual difference" (64). The bodily and discursive rupture created by transsexuality is how Iranian transsexuals perform their subjectivity.

Be Like Others and the Ethics of Representation in Documentary

Be Like Others (in Persian/Farsi with English titles and subtitles) is a Western-produced documentary directed by U.S.-based Iranian filmmaker, Tanaz Eshaghian.[6] The film follows the narratives of several male to female transsexuals (MtF) including 20-year-old Anoosh, 25-year-old Ali Askar, and 26-year-old Farhad (Ali Askar's friend). There are also some accounts from the post-op MtF Vida and other transsexuals who come to the Mirdamad Surgical Center.

The meticulous selection of Iranian transsexuals for the film contributes to an engaging narrative. The film uses direct interviews as its main documentary technique and does not have any narration or voice-over. Also, the viewer does not hear the interviewer's questions, except in some occasions. In fact, the characters' responses reveal the nature of the questions. Eshaghian's technical approach creates two paradoxical contexts in the film. First, the absence of the filmmaker from the screen does not simply work toward the subjectification of Iranian transsexuals in the film by giving them more visual and discursive presence. Instead, as the interview questions typically reference the illegality of homosexuality in the country, the filmmaker's perspective is constantly foregrounded. For instance, in a scene in which the question is not heard, Vida explains her view of homosexuality:

VIDA: (responding to the interviewer): When someone is really male, feel that they are male, yet they use "alternative" ways sexually, I don't approve of such behavior.
INTERVIEWER: What don't you like?
VIDA: These gay individuals that you mentioned.

This conversation points to the constructedness of the film's perspective based on the filmmaker's vision, and highlights the ethics associated with this construction of reality. As Bill Nichols asserts, "The presence (and absence) of the filmmaker in the image, in off-screen space, in the acoustic folds of voice-on and voice-off, in titles and graphics constitutes an ethics, and a politics, of considerable importance to the viewer" (Representing Reality 77). He names this ethical matter "axiographics," which "address[es] the question of how values, particularly an ethics of representation, comes to be known and experienced in relation to space" (77). In the mentioned scene, the interviewer/filmmaker should have considered the fact that publicly acknowledging homosexuality in Iran can be problematic for the interviewee, given the illegality and religious unacceptability associated with it in the country—ironically this is the point that the filmic narrative constantly reminds us—and therefore, Vida as a post-op transsexual living in Iran might not be able to express her opinion explicitly.[7]

The persistent reference to homosexuality in *Be Like Others* attempts to undermine the acceptance of transsexuality in Iran as an Islamic country. Elhum Shakerifar explains that "the use of stereotypical images of Tehran given constantly in the film serves to heighten the controversy that was introduced in the opening statements of the film" (335). The juxtaposition of transsexual subjects—the interviewees—with images of a mosque, clerics, and veiled women in Tehran all serve to enforce a conservative interpretation of Iran and underestimate its religious and legal acceptance of transsexuality. However, the consideration of transsexuality not only as a sexual transition, but also as a psychic and social movement provides a counter-narrative to this reductive illustration.

Transsexual Transition and Spatial Transgression

In "Of Other Spaces: Utopias and Heterotopias" Michel Foucault observes, "[W]e do not live in a sort of a vacuum, within which individuals and things can be located ... but in a set of relationships that define positions which cannot be equated or in any way superimposed" (351). These relationships form power relations, hierarchies, margins, and the Other. The coming out of Iranian transsexuals can trouble the configuration of social spaces that are shaped based on gender-segregation laws and are constantly policed and regulated.[8] Thus, the consideration of these spaces becomes important in discussing the formation of transsexual identity and subjectivity in Iran. I distinguish three spaces—public (society), private (family), and medical (clinic)—that are governed by the state in one way or another, in addition to a filmic space formed by the intrusion of the camera within these contested spaces.

Social and Familial Spaces

As the accounts of interviewees in *Be Like Others* show, transsexuality is considered an explicit challenge to gender-segregated boundaries creating slippages that can threaten the sexual politics of the Iranian state.

VIDA: When I was a boy, I had too many problems out there. ... If I walked on the street either the police, the Revolutionary Guard, or the Morality Police would arrest me. ... They would take me and disrespect me badly.

ALI: (the boyfriend of MtF Anoosh): I'd like you to see what it's like walking down the street with him[/her]. Ninety percent of people we pass say something nasty. ... My biggest problem is with the people around us.

There are two main points in these accounts. First, the discourse of power in Iranian society is enacted not only by the state, but also by some citizens who normalize their society, internalizing the regulatory, heteronormative laws. Second, in the case of MtF transsexuals, the tangible change of spatial mobility comes to the fore as they adapt to female gender roles which in Iranian society are often defined through the domestication of the female body. For both pre-op and post-op MtF transsexuals, thus, the identification process partly comes through the significant change of mobility within public and domestic spaces and performativity within each space. This performance is depicted in a scene in which Anoosh goes to the Police Station to obtain a written "permit" allowing him/her to easily commute in public spaces as a transsexual, especially in regard to his/her hijab.

DISTRICT POLICE ATTORNEY: I will give you a letter so that you won't have problems. ... But ... while it's true that you're stuck between genders, your body moves like a female. So, you will have to follow the Islamic laws for females.

ANOOSH: Definitely! I have to completely respect the limitations placed on a woman.

DISTRICT POLICE ATTORNEY: They are not limitations.

ANOOSH: Yes, but the freedom I had as a boy, I'll never have as a girl. Right? I could wear short sleeves or whatever else, but as a girl, I won't be doing such things. I know all of this. I'm trying to get used to it.

This lament highlights the compulsory restrictions imposed upon Iranian women in the name of sexual difference, and also points to the performativity of gender constructions. As Judith Butler writes in regard to gender performance, "Gender is the repeated stylization of the body, a set of repeated acts within a highly rigid regulatory frame that congeal over time to produce the appearance of substance, of a natural sort of being" (*Gender Trouble* 45). In the context of Iranian society, this becoming is not limited to the realm of personal or private, rather it embodies the politics of power relations that normalizes transsexual existence through documentation, and points to the instability of gender-segregated social boundaries. The state-issued forms and medical documents themselves are proof of the constructedness of gender and its performativity. The transition of Iranian transsexuals, therefore, should not be read as a linear movement as the film suggests, but rather as a complex process of multiple transformations that are constantly in negotiation with the volatile sexual politics of the state.

In *Be Like Others* the private space of the family paradoxically works both as an extension of the controlled public space, mirroring traditional socio-cultural norms and regulating the visibility and mobility of the transsexual body, and also as a space where transsexuals can freely express themselves and perform their identities. The recognition of personal and social identity is firmly tied to the place of each person within the familial structure. For example, Ali Askar's family ostracizes him/her because of his/her transsexuality. The traumatic and devastating consequences of this ostracization loom in Ali Askar's life while s/he attempts to focus on the re-construction of his/her identity through SRS. Farhad (Ali Askar's friend) also laments, "It's afterwards I worry about. Our families will officially disown us after the operation. It's painful. This is just the beginning of hell." In this situation, aside from having emotional and psychological effects, a family's denunciation can shatter the transsexual's social recognition.

Familial pressures on Iranian transsexuals find their roots in a cultural tradition of recognizing a male/female binary as the only model of sexual and gender identity. Enforcing this notion on transsexuals, thus, can be read as a performative extension of the state's heterosexual ideology. Anoosh, for instance, before SRS, experiences a certain freedom and mobility at home, especially in terms of his/her relationship with boyfriend Ali. Anoosh's mother emphasizes that Anoosh can use make up and wear any women's dress at home. However, after SRS, Anoosh is subject to stricter scrutiny as a woman. As sexual and intimate relationships of unrelated men and women in Iran are not religiously or socially acceptable, Anoosh's mother insists that their association be legally and officially documented through marriage. Although the extent to which Iranian transsexuals position their relations to the heteronormative rules varies, conforming to them after SRS is mostly based on the transsexuals' need for a social and personal sense of security and acceptance within both social and familial spaces.

Medical and Filmic Spaces

Dr. Mir-Jalali, one of the leading surgeons of sex-change operation in Iran, in a conversation with a FtM transsexual, featured in *Be Like Others*, says, "I cannot turn you into a complete, full male. You won't be able to reproduce. You cannot make a family. Physically, you will not achieve the prowess and virility of Tarzan." The medical discourse of incompleteness and abnormality, practiced here, defines transsexuality through its comparison with the constructed body types (male/female) and their "realness." In this context, the visible surface of the body such as sex organs, breasts, facial hair, and so on sets the norm for defining gender identity. As Foucault in this regard points out, "[T]he clinic appears—in terms of the doctor's experience—as a new outline of the perceptible and statable: a new distribution of the discrete elements of corporal space" (The Birth of the Clinic xviii). The medical discourse, thus, underlines the essentialist notion of sexual difference and puts itself in alignment with the heterosexual ideology of the Iranian state.

The medical notion of transsexuality in Iran aptly distinguishes between transsexuality and homosexuality. The supportive argument in this regard, however, seems problematic because it emphasizes the willingness of transsexuals to undergo SRS as something that does not pertain to homosexuals. In this context, SRS is viewed as a bodily transformation that matches the body with the psyche and creates a tangible gender identity based on a heteronormative structure. Dr. Mir-Jalali mentions, "A homosexual is never willing to operate. ... I give such a difficult and terrible description [of SRS] that a homosexual runs out of [my office] by the third sentence. ... A transsexual says, 'That's my desire!'" In fact, the process of sex change in Iran, which operates based on various governmental and medical documents, such as psychological reports, blood and hormonal tests, and governmental permission for SRS (in order to allow a transsexual to obtain a new birth certificate after operation), echoes the Foucauldian concept of the "medical gaze," aiming to define and construct transsexual identity through a stack of reports and visible evidence: "The eye becomes the depositary and source of clarity; it has the power to bring a truth to light that it receives only to the extent that it has brought it to light" (*The Birth of the Clinic* xiii). The medical gaze in the film in particular shows itself in the scenes that focus on Ali Askar's SRS. In a scene in which Ali Askar is resting on a bed in the hospital after his/her sex-change operation, Dr. Mir-Jalali's colleague enters the room and examines Ali Askar's belly by pressing his hand on it. A trace of pain appears on Ali Askar's face, but the doctor, looking into the camera, says, "I stitched up [her belly] myself. Come see how marvelous it is!" The impression of a successful operation, embodied through good-looking stitches, contradicts the pain experienced by Ali Askar, and connects itself to the paradoxical state of a fully transitioned, and yet, inauthentic body within a heteronormative context that an Iranian transsexual should face after his/her sex-change operation.

The medical gaze and its limitation of capturing the truth can be read in comparison to the filmic gaze in documentary film: "As an anthropomorphic extension of the human sensorium the camera reveals not only the world but its operator's preoccupations, subjectivity, and values" (Nichols, *Representing Reality* 79). Thus, there is no doubt that like the medical gaze, the scope of the filmic gaze is also limited and mediated. Particularly in ethnographic and anthropological documentary films, the camera can record what is on the surface and actually can be seen, which "means that many of the intricacies involved in cultural practices escape the lens, owing to the minimal scope of actuality footage or the intrusion of the camera" (Mathew 20). Regarding documentary films on transsexual lives, the extent of the camera intrusion is highly sensitive as it may risk fetishizing the transsexual body, taking away transsexual subjectivity, and/or creating identification between transsexual subject and viewer through sympathy.

In the case of *Be Like Others* the fetishization comes from the neo-Orientalist discursive process of Othering, which aims to understand the issues of Iranian transsexuals in an Islamic country within the context of homosexuality. This approach ignores the complexity of the formation of transsexual identity in Iran to foreground conservatism associated with its society. As Behdad and Williams assert, "Orientalism always entails rearticulations of otherness to ensure its cultural hegemony in the face of complex political and social change" (298). There is no doubt that the Iranian-American nationality of the filmmaker plays a fundamental role in allowing her to enter the private and familial spaces of Iranian transsexuals. Eshaghian's Iranian background creates a trust that seemingly blurs the boundaries of "they" versus "us," engendering some intimate and personal responses and reactions from the transsexual interviewees and their friends and families. However, the constructed rhetoric of the film from the beginning breaks the moments of filmic intimacy by imposing the filmmaker's perspective on the subjects, and therefore, on the film's structure. Nonetheless, the transsexual characters in the film represent their agency through constant negotiations with regulatory norms within social, familial, and medical spaces, at the same time subverting the Western stereotypes of passivity and victimhood in an Islamic country.

Toward the end of the film, the title "One Year Later," announces temporal, spatial, and sexual changes in the lives of the characters. Following Anoosh's, Ali Askar's, and Farhad's stories through this passage of time, the viewer further recognizes the complexity of the formation of transsexual identity and subjectivity in Iranian society as each of them has chosen or has been forced to follow a different path in his/her life. Anoosh has now fully transitioned to a woman (Anahita) and is engaged to Ali. Although she is completely satisfied with her status as a woman, the cultural and social norms governing the segregated lives of men and women in Iran have problematized her relationship with Ali. Ali Askar has also fully transitioned to a woman (Negar) and lives with some transsexual friends in Tehran. As she explains to the camera, after SRS her family shunned her. Going through a period of depression, she now likes her "new world." Negar further mentions that she works as a sex worker and points to the dark side of the lives of some post-op transsexuals in Iran, who regardless of their transition, cannot fit into the social and familial spaces and continue to live on the margins of the society. As Negar says, "Since we do not have female reproductive parts and cannot get pregnant, we can get [temporarily] married ... We are selling our bodies. We are not selling our souls." According to Iranian religious discourse on transsexuality, SRS is supposed to match the body with the soul. Negar's statement, however, points to the idea that for her, the body is still detached. The body was not authentic before and it is not now. This detachment allows Negar to subvert the expectations of chastity and domesticity that define her new gender and to perform her subjectivity at the margins. Farhad, on the other hand, has put a halt to his/her SRS and lives as a transsexual in a permanent state of "transition." S/he explains various difficulties that have happened to his/her transsexual friends after their sex-change operation, such as suicidal thoughts, sexual incompetence, and physical and mental problems. Farhad in this regard says, "I want to have a decent life. Be like others. [But] when I saw all of these things, I decided to hold off because I don't want my life to get worse." It is this non-conformity to a specific sexual category (male/female) and staying in the transition phase that give Farhad his/her subjectivity. The fact that regardless of his/her uneasy mobility within various spaces, Farhad decides to remain a transsexual presents the performativity of his/her agency in addition to his/her gender performance. These various performances and subjectivities of Iranian transsexuals remind us that the readings and/or representations of transsexuality in Iran (or any other country) need to be attuned to the complexity of the society and the multiplicity of legal, cultural, religious, and medical discourses pertinent to the context. It is with this consideration that a non-biased, comprehensive, and multi-dimensional understanding of transsexuality can be achieved. An issue that regardless of an urgent topic and an engaging filmic narrative is underestimated in Tanaz Eshaghian's *Be Like Others*.

Notes

1 For example, *Yellow Cruise* (1934), directed by Leon Poirier, shows the horse-drawn street cars in Tehran, which was negatively received by Iranians living abroad and Iranian intellectuals inside Iran as a showcase of "a backward country" (Naficy 219).
2 Behdad and Williams further argue that while "predominantly a North American phenomenon, neo-Orientalism is not limited to the United States; nor is it merely produced by Western subjects. On the contrary, not only do Middle Eastern writers,

scholars, and so-called experts participate in its production, but they play an active and significant role in propagating it" (284).

3 See also Niloufar Haidari's reflection on the Western-centric and Orientalist approach of the documentary film *Raving Iran* (2016), directed by Susanne Regina Meures, at https://noisey.vice.com/en_us/article/ywbnab/raving-iran-film-documentary-blade-beard.

4 Katarzyna Korycki and Abouzar Nasirzadeh discuss the nuances of the Iranian state's approach to homosexuality in "the last two hundred years in Iran," observing that "far from being the pawn of Western machinations, the Iranian state has varied its stance toward homosexuality in pursuit of its objectives – namely modernization, consolidation, and most recently, deliberalization. ... To achieve these objectives, it first borrowed an anti-homosexual stance from the West, only to later claim homosexuality itself was a Western import" (174).

5 Afsaneh Najmabadi highlights that, "[w]hen it comes to sex change, as with many other issues, there is no unanimity of opinion among Shi'i scholars who issue fatwas in Iran. All consider intersex surgeries permissible because they bring out 'the hidden genus' of the body. Some explicitly argue against non-intersex surgeries, while others express doubt about its permissibility or simply do not take a stand. ... Regardless of these differing stances, it was the overwhelming weight of Ayatollah Khomeini's fatwa that translated into law" (*Professing Selves* 174).

6 "Born in Iran in 1974, Eshaghian emigrated to the United States shortly after the 1979 revolution. ... For *Be Like Others*, her début feature-length film, Eshaghian returned to Iran for the first time in 25 years" (ITVS).

7 Afsaneh Najmabadi explains that the separation of transsexuality from homosexuality, which is usually considered a moral deviation in various Iranian discourses, has provided a means for the legitimation of trans identity and the acceptability of trans individuals in society: "This is also why so many trans persons, at least in publicized domains, say, ever insistently, 'we are not same-sex-players.' It has become a grid of self-cognition through dis-identification" (*Professing Selves* 248).

8 Najmeh Moradiyan-Rizi in this regard writes, "In today's Iran, the authority of the Islamic state over the Iranian women's bodies explicitly shows itself in the establishment of 'Moral[ity] Police.' The Moral[ity] Police appears on streets of Iranian cities and monitors the veiling of Iranian women according to its own Islamic criteria. If a woman does not meet the criteria, she will be fined or condemned to prison" (23).

Works Cited

Behdad, Ali. *Camera Orientalis: Reflections on Photography of the Middle East*. Chicago: U of Chicago P, 2016.

Behdad, Ali and Juliet Williams. "Neo-Orientalism." *Globalizing American Studies*. Ed. Brian T. Edwards and Dilip Parameshwar Gaonkar. Chicago: U of Chicago P, 2010. 283–299.

Bucar, Elizabeth and Anne Enke. "Unlikely Sex Change Capitals of the World: Trinidad, United States, and Tehran, Iran, as Twin Yardsticks of Homonormative Liberalism." *Feminist Studies* 37. 2(2011): 301–328.

Butler, Judith. "Critically Queer." *GLQ: A Journal of Lesbian and Gay Studies* 1. 1 (1993): 17–32.

Butler, Judith. *Gender Trouble: Feminism and the Subversion of Identity*. New York: Routledge, 2006.

Foucault, Michel. *The Birth of the Clinic: An Archaeology of Medical Perception*. Trans. A.M. Sheridan Smith. New York: Pantheon Books, 1973.

Foucault, Michel. "Of Other Spaces: Utopias and Heterotopias." *Rethinking Architecture: A Reader in Cultural Theory.* Ed. Neil Leach. New York: Routledge, 1997. 350–356.

Hamedani, Ali. "The Gay People Pushed to Change Their Gender." *BBC News,* 5 November 2014. www.bbc.com/news/magazine-29832690.

ITVS. *Be Like Others.* https://itvs.org/films/be-like-others.

Kamali Dehghan, Saeed. "Iran's Persecution of Gay Community Revealed." *The Guardian,* 17 May 2012. www.theguardian.com/world/2012/may/17/iran-persecution-gay-community-revealed.

Korycki, Katarzyna and Abouzar Nasirzadeh. "Homophobia as a Tool of Statecraft: Iran and Its Queers." *Global Homophobia: States, Movements, and the Politics of Oppression.* Ed. Meredith L. Weiss and Michael J. Bosia. Urbana: U of Illinois P, 2013. 174–195.

Littauer, Dan. "Iran Performed over 1,000 Gender Reassignment Operations in Four Years." *Gay Star News,* 4 December 2012. www.gaystarnews.com/article/iran-performed-over-1000-gender-reassignment-operations-four-years041212/.

Mathew, Wesley. "Reality in Ethnographic Film: Documentary vs. Docudrama." *Visual Anthropology* 27(2014): 17–24.

Moradiyan-Rizi, Najmeh. "Iranian Women, Iranian Cinema: Negotiating with Ideology and Tradition." *Journal of Religion and Film* 19.1(2015): Article 35.

Naficy, Hamid. "Nonfiction Fiction: Documentaries on Iran." *Iranian Studies* 12. 3/4 (1979): 217–238.

Nagel, Joane. "Ethnicity and Sexuality." *Annual Review of Sociology* 26(2000): 107–133.

Najmabadi, Afsaneh. *Professing Selves: Transsexuality and Same-Sex Desire in Contemporary Iran.* Durham: Duke UP, 2014.

Najmabadi, Afsaneh. "Transing and Transpassing across Sex-Gender Walls in Iran." *Women's Studies Quarterly* 36. 3/4 (2008): 23–42.

Nichols, Bill. *Introduction to Documentary.* Bloomington: Indiana UP, 2001.

Nichols, Bill. *Representing Reality: Issues and Concepts in Documentary.* Bloomington: Indiana UP, 1991.

Oldershausen, Sasha von. "Iran's Sex-Change Operations Provided Nearly Free-Of-Cost." *The Huffington Post,* 4 June, 2012. www.huffingtonpost.com/2012/06/04/iran-sex-change-operation_n_1568604.html.

Prosser, Jay. *Second Skins: The Body Narratives of Transsexuality.* New York: Columbia UP, 1998.

Scott, Joan W. "Feminism's History." *Journal of Women's History* 16. 2(2004): 10–29.

Shakerifar, Elhum. "Visual Representations of Iranian Transgenders." *Iranian Studies* 44. 3(2011): 327–339.

6   Isolated Bodies, Isolated Spaces

Anorexia and Bulimia in Women's Autobiographical Narratives

Barbara Grüning

Introduction

Thinness as an expression of individual success offers a simple explanation for the need for self-control through the body (Ostuzzi and Luxardi). "Pro-ana" groups on social media treat anorexia as a superior ethos and lifestyle choice (Boero and Pascoe) and thereby perfectly synthesize the idea that the "society of the spectacle" (Debord) has a direct influence on the onset of anorexia or other eating disorders like bulimia. However, this example runs the risk of reducing the contemporary phenomenon of anorexia to a new media event, when its roots can be traced back much further. This chapter considers the spatial perceptions, experiences, and representations of the body in twenty-one autobiographic narratives by Italian women with anorexia, bulimia, or both in the past three decades.[1] The social and cultural environments of southern and northern Italian cities, the influence of Italian Catholic culture on gender roles, the authors' social status and the historical context (Di Viggiano and Bufano; Maione) significantly shape both the women's spatial experience of their body and the ways this experience is narrated. In this regard, I will distinguish among three types of narrative structure (Robson), which correspond to three different emotional styles.

   The first type of autobiography follows the model of the diary, which some anorexic/bulimic women began for therapeutic purposes. The narratives mainly focus on these women's life in eating disorder centers and describe a period of maximum five years, with some flashbacks to the life before the onset of anorexia (Bandoli; Guizzetti; Brunello; Artemisia; Grazioli; Miglietta, Boero; Cobainsbaby). As a result, they describe eating and further cultural practices as influenced by the spatial-temporal norms of the hospital's institutionalized spaces: the panic before and after being weighed; the irritation with some hospital rules; the boredom felt in the empty time between compulsory meals, the defiance towards the medical staff, and the rare moments of cheer with other anorexic and/or bulimic patients. Authors of this type of autobiography possess a "high institutionalized cultural capital" and/or a "high embodied cultural capital" (cf. Bourdieu, "The Forms of Capital"), with the exception of Bandoli and Grazioli. Even though the social world outside the hospital is largely relegated to the background, the authors nevertheless offer some interesting clues about it and all reject the bourgeois values with which they grew up.

The second type of autobiography retraces the negative episodes experienced by the authors from their childhood to the present (De Clercq; Bruni; Sabbadini; Gardino; Pasquadibisceglie; La Bella; Strappafelci). These autobiographies share some distinctive characteristics: anorexia is a chronic disease and remembering the past life before the onset of anorexia is useful to reinterpret the current condition as originating from difficult familial relationships. Furthermore, the emotions are expressed with more naivety and intensity than in the first group of autobiographies. It seems that the emotional grammar these women learnt as children in the family context is inadequate to express what they really feel. Most of these authors originated from the lower-middle class (Bruni; Sabbadini; Pasquadibisceglie; Strappafelci), except for De Clercq and they grew up either in country areas in southern and central Italy (La Bella and Gardino) or in the peripheries and hinterlands of (industrial) big cities such as Rome, Turin, and Milan. The parents' social expectations relegate the daughters to the kitchen, evidencing the endurance of a patriarchal family model.

The third type of autobiography presents a nonlinear narrative structure. Within this type, there are two kinds of narratives: those which weave together episodes of the past, imaginary dialogues with "significant others" (Mead), and long descriptions of bodily sensations (Tangheri; Gamberale); and those which aim at using the author's own painful experiences to reflect on some broader question, such as the difficulties for women of having a career and the gendered structure of society (Arachi; Longo; Marzano; Vaniglia Orelli). In the first case the anorexic experience is mediated by a poetic and metaphoric style of writing, in the second case by an ironic and reflective one. As a result, the narrative structure and style create an emotional distance from the suffering the authors felt during their illness. The authors in this group all belong to the upper intellectual class, with the exception of Longo.

Psychoanalytic and Feminist Approaches to Anorexia

Scientific discourse originally framed anorexia and bulimia psychoanalytically, as eating disorders or mental illnesses resulting from disturbed mother–daughter relationships. Thomas and Marikai Vander Ven noted that just after WWII, self-starvation episodes were interpreted as a carryover of a mother's inability to feed daughters during childhood. During adolescence, these disturbed eating patterns continued, simultaneously suppressing budding sexual impulses (Alpert; Sperling). In the 1960s and 1970s, object-relations theory based on analyses of parent–child communication portrayed mothers who discouraged autonomy and self-expression as the main cause of anorexia (Crisp, "Psychological Aspect"; Malagoli Togliatti). Self-starvation was a way for young girls to separate from the mother and protect their egos (Selvini Palazzoli). By the eighties, anorexia began to be analyzed through a systems model that presented family as not the cause, but rather the context, for anorexia. According to

Minuchin et al. contrasting social expectations at work and in traditional female roles caused anorexia. Meanwhile, feminist scholars (Orbach, "Accepting the Symptom"; Goode) attributed anorexia to patriarchal culture, leading to a growing inclusion of sociocultural explanations in psychoanalytic interpretations. In these models, however, society often appears as an abstract entity that exercises deterministic power over anorexic women.

Subsequent psychoanalytic interpretations see anorexia as both a symptom and consequence of a narcissistic culture, characteristic of hypermodern reality (Recalcati). Just as narcissistic subjects continually reject others, anorexic subjects reject the body as the place of "the other." In this interpretation, anorexic bodies close in on themselves: a *"false self"* corresponds to a *"false body"* (Orbach, Hunger Strike) and is "fashioned as a narcissistic defense against threatening exteriority" (Bray and Colebrook 52). Feminist scholars (Bray and Colebrook; Malson), however, criticize the correspondence between false self and false body as resting upon a Cartesian body/mind dualism that casts women as passive entities who unconsciously assimilate social discourses. According to Judith Butler, women perform gender to produce "a set of corporeal styles" (524) that may not be culturally proscribed. Feminist sociologist Morag MacSween observes that women "try to synthesize their social position through the creation of the 'anorexic body'" (2), which can also be seen as a response to women's identity being reduced to female sexuality. Self-starvation shapes the body into a neutral form to signify *non-gendered subjectivity*. In particular MacSween raises three objections to a psychoanalytic interpretation of anorexia: the assumption that culture is external to the individual (Slade), which implies that the practices of anorexic women are not socially constructed; the idea that "anorexia rests on the concept of the 'integrated body self' or 'ego synthesis'" (MacSween 42; Bruch), which requires a static conception of the body; and the fact that psychiatric approaches to eating disorders are based on predefined notions of "normal" that inevitably lead to classifying anorexics as "abnormal" (Crisp, Anorexia Nervosa). In contrast, recent social science approaches stress the need to de-medicalize anorexic events (Rich; O'Connor and Van Esterik; Darmon, "The Fifth Element"). Separating social discourses on anorexia from anorexics' experiences shows that medicalization cannot always decode the cultural meanings in anorexic stories and lives.

From Gendered Spaces to Anorexic Spaces

The 1990s saw a broader social science and feminist perspective not only to anorexia, but also to space and its relationship to gender (Duncan). In *Space, Place and Gender* (1994), geographer Doreen Massey identifies space as shaped materially and discursively through social interactions. Dichotomous classifications like public/private reflect historically male ideology, which produces symbolic and social boundaries between places for women and men that correspond to different scripts of practices, interactions, and behaviors. Angela McRobbie argues that the modern patriarchal symbolic order is decentralized, disseminated and untraceable, making it more complicated for women to identify gendered power structures in everyday life. Indeed, as Elisabeth Grosz points out, "it is our positioning within space, both as the point of perspectival access to space, and also an object for others in space, that gives the subject a coherent identity and ability to manipulate things, including its own bodies parts, in space" (19). What happens, however, when a body appears incongruous because it invades "the normative location of body in space" (Puwar 52)?

Two implications of the feminist work on space are important here from a phenomenological viewpoint. First, personal spatializing practices (Löw, Raum-soziologie) modify relational spaces even for subjects trying to make their presence invisible or those who are socially and culturally invisible to others. For instance, the autobiographic narratives of anorexic/bulimic women show how they try to reduce their own physical bodies, while also trying to draw attention to them. Ironically, higher visibility as "non-normative bodies" leads anorexic women to withdraw from public spaces. Being labeled as "anorexic" generates not only a sense of shame but also a feeling of isolation despite the presence of other interacting bodies and subjectivities in the same space. This dynamic of identity stripping is especially evident within peer groups, as Cobainsbaby writes when she describes her return to school after a period in an eating disorder center: "For them I was 'that anorexic' and no longer 'Elena.' They were like vultures waiting for the death of their prey" (Cobainsbaby 82–83). Second is the idea of the body as a territory with a line "drawn around it" (Irigaray 17). In the autobiographies I reviewed, anorexic/bulimic women reinforce the line between their body and the external world mostly in two ways: by refusing foods as symbolic mediation with the external world and by restricting progressively their (material) space of life, so that it can contain only their anorexic bodies. This process consists of three steps: anorexic women refrain from entering public urban spaces; they refuse to live in the convivial spaces of their home, such as the kitchen and the living room, where food is prepared or consumed together, and they confine themselves to their bed.

Caruana noticed that "the anorexic has some personal semantic space of her own," which "may be described in existentialist terms as a form of self-realization" (182). Anorexic individuals build their semantic space to reject a common language in a linguistic sense, and also, in a broader cultural sense, the shared forms of sensory, symbolic, and corporeal interaction (Knoblauch and Löw). Hence, the ways anorexic women try to re-structure physical and rela-tional spaces through their bodies (Moss and Dyck) incorporate a language of non-normative practices that govern their routines with other bodies (Bray and Colebrook).

The structure of power relationships among agents with different social posi-tions—the extent and composition of their social, economic, and cultural resour-ces—should also be considered (Bourdieu, *Distinction*). Darmon examines how class position socially conditions the "possibility of an anorexic career" ("The Fifth Element" 718) that does not exclude, as the autobiographies highlight, lower social classes as it reworks values, principles, and tastes of the middle-upper class such as corporeal asceticism as a form of elitism. Following Darmon, I consider an *anorexic habitus*, [2] an internal disposition constituted by a set of repeated practices that structures the everyday lives of anorexics, by which the body becomes a "vector of knowledge of social world" (Wacquant 88; Silva). The anorexic habitus is formed by different yet deeply-interlaced practices: *food anorexic practices*, aimed at reducing and transforming corporeal space; and *relational anorexic practices*, or the pragmatic daily problem of managing the anorexic body in both private and public spaces. Both sets of practices control body space and imply a "non-normative" perception of social and relational spaces, highlighting two apparently conflicting spatial processes. Anorexic women reinforce corporeal boundaries to separate themselves from social and relational spaces, while simultaneously trying to mask their condition in public and continue their everyday practices, at least until they are able to support this duality.

Darmon distinguishes four phases of an anorexic career. First, anorexics decide to go on a diet, then, by systematically repeating practices aimed at losing weight, they structure an anorexic habitus. The third phase is characterized by "discretion" and "illusion work" aimed at making anorexic practices less perceptible ("The Fifth Element" 722). The fourth stage or "hospital phase" offers a solution to the duality of anorexics' lives through detachment from normal life. This stage is characterized by the resistance to the role of patient under medical control. Of course, some anorexic women are never hospitalized while others are hospitalized multiple times. Thus, the "anorexic career" model is only heuristic and not universally applicable.

Too Much Weight: A Spatial Question

By questioning their biological and social existence, anorexics and bulimics develop and put into practice a peculiar idea of space, departing from their own mental and physical spaces (Parr and Butler). As one author writes about her illness: "anorexia is the extreme symbolic challenge to the biological limit of one's own body" (Vaniglia Orelli 104). The enduring desire to "feel empty" (Artemisia 33; Arachi 17) can be actualized either by reducing the quantity of food taken into the body or by vomiting. To realize these two fundamental practices, anorexic/bulimic women construct a mental map of real places where their practices are invisible, or successful, and places where they are exposed to others, and therefore lose control:

> I went outside and ran to the bar to eat cookies and sandwiches … I also found a place where I could throw up the food before going back home. It was a sleazy little garden with only three completely broken wooden benches. At night this little garden was dark, half-hidden, and used to the vomit of drunk people, the wrappers of the homeless, the syringes, and the empty boxes of condoms.
>
> (Arachi 78–79)

Anorexic/bulimic women progressively retreat from social situations and relational spaces which threaten their mind and body space:

I should pay attention to my friends, limit the physical and mental proximity to others, and avoid intimate moments and the risks of being discovered for what I felt to be a life-long mistake.

(Sabbadini 55)

In this regard, the decision to be confined within institutionalized spaces such as the hospital upholds the possibility of openly displaying one's illness, since these places structure their everyday lives as "non-normal" (Turner):

It is not possible to hold glassware or any other sharp objects such as razor blades, tweezers, mirrors, lamps and so on. It is also forbidden to lock the door of the restroom and of the bedroom. ... You have to wake up at 8.30, have breakfast at 9.00, have lunch at 12.30, and have dinner at 7.00 p.m. You have to eat with others in a common room. In short, this was the place where I was.

(Cobainsbaby 29)

Another point of interest is that in the majority of the autobiographies,[3] the women see anorexia as an outside element occupying a space in their body. Anorexia is personified as another "living, thinking subject" that occupies one's mind and controls bodily actions: a "bloody beast," "monster," "foul being," "vampire," "wicked viper," "filthy being," "cancer of the soul"[4] or a "new creature," "best friend," or "female voice jealous of one's friends" (Arachi; Artemisia; Boero; Cobainsbaby; De Clercq; Gamberale; Guizzetti; La Bella; Marzano; Sabbadini; Strappafelci; Tangheri). However, attempts to materially define anorexia point at a lack of clear contours, "something black, heavy and thick" (Cobainsbaby 98). Over time, these women find it increasingly difficult to delimit the spaces of anorexia or bulimia: the interior world seems boundless, and the fine line between mind and body disappears. Anorexia progressively conquers new spaces, devouring "pieces of oneself" (Cobainsbaby 133) until the capability to feel is lost. Following Darmon's phases, despite initial happiness at controlling the body, after an anorexic habitus is consolidated the women recognize this as only the "happiness of the beast" (Guizzetti). Their feelings become "anesthetized" (La Bella) until their senses can no longer mediate between internal and external worlds, the gaze is absent (Arachi; Guizzetti), the voices of others are perceived only as noises (De Clercq), and there is no more interest in physical contact (Grazioli).

As anorexia or bulimia progresses, women experience conflicts between what they consider the sane, normal part and the sick, non-normal parts of themselves. However, sanity belongs more to memory than a present divided between hidden ritual practices, such as not eating, throwing up, constantly weighing oneself, chopping food, measuring calories, obsessive physical exercise, as well as practices aimed at hiding one's physical and mental state. These women can no longer continue their usual activities of studying, working, reading, painting, going to parties or pubs (Sabbadini). At first, they believe that reinforcing self-control and autonomy over food will strengthen their public lives and hence their symbolic power (Warin), yet progressively the fear of being discovered leads anorexic women to retreat and reduce the space of their lives. Parallel to this transformation of practices and spaces, a sense of identity also changes; while anorexia initially constructs a new identity independent from social confirmations and judgments, it later prevents social relationships with the outside world.

Anorexic/bulimic women use metaphors to describe their body shift during the different phases of their anorexic careers. Initially, the desire to feel as light as a butterfly (Marzano; La Bella) gives some women a sense of independence, especially from their family. Being empty represents the possibility to define one's own space through the body (Sabbadini). The "four bones" of the hips are the form and involucre of this personal space (La Bella). Touching these bones, a frequent gesture, provides reassurance of the solidity of a corporeal barrier that prevents external things and subjects from penetrating internal space (Sabbadini; Vaniglia Orelli). The body becomes a "provisory container" (De Clercq), traversed not only by food but also all social meanings and relationships. The transformation of the body through anorexic/bulimic practices also objectifies the social world. Spaces and places are considered only insofar as they function for ritualized practices (i.e. the public or private restroom for vomiting). The anorexic body continues *to stay* in the social world but in a fixed, inaccessible corporeal space. However, by refusing to interact with other bodies, anorexic women deny themselves the chance to negotiate the structure of meanings underlying social spaces. In public spaces, the recognition and consequent vulnerability of an anorexic body increases (Cobainsbaby; Arachi).

The corporeal barrier, the protruding bones, give the anorexic woman the impression of strengthening her autonomy and protecting the "suffering" that she treasures in her body space from others (La Bella; Guizzetti; Cobainsbaby). Reducing her own existential space becomes a strategy for protecting herself from the outside world:

> I retreat into myself on my little cloud and I stopped looking down. There was nothing I was interested of seeing, they can do what they want with me. I would have limited myself to disappear, to reduce the surface of my body, so that those who wanted to rough me would have had difficulty finding my body.
>
> (Sabbadini 87)

> My idea, my brilliant project was to flip through my limbs, one layer at a time, and to see in every removed piece of flesh a piece of grief going away forever.
>
> (Vaniglia Orelli 41–42)

Independent of original causes (for example, rape), the separation of the body from the external world progressively loses any concrete reference and significance. Therefore, anorexics feel a "sense of emptiness" they then project onto the external world. Ultimately, the only solution seems to be a further reduction of the corporeal space, so they "are able to grasp with their own hands, to envelop" their own bodies (Guizzetti 196). Clothing protects by masking the body from others (Arachi) and preserving a symbolic physical distance (Gamberale). In the end, the bedroom and bed remain[5] the last refuge for a body, separated from other familiar spaces that incorporate family tensions (Sabbadini).

The hospital or the center for eating disorders may be negatively experienced as a form of total control over oneself (Goffman). However, these experiences differ basically according to the social status of the woman. Women with little cultural (institutional and embodied) capital—in the Bourdieuian sense—are unable to escape the rigid doctor–patient relationship spatialized in hospitals (Sabbadini; Grazioli; Pasquadibisceglie; La Bella), since they are less able to appropriate and manage (also emotionally) certain values and attitudes which they never incorporated. The medical staff exercises authoritarian forms of knowledge, deriving from their expertise, which are unintelligible to these women:

> The staff seemed made of ice, cold, and detached. Everything I thought and said was an expression and symptom of a pathology.
>
> (La Bella 40)

The staff's behavior increases the perception that hospitals are cold and unfamiliar places where anorexic and bulimic women are crushed: "locked up in a super-prison which is instead a super-clinic" (Sabbatini 107; see also Bruni 83 and Pasquadibisceglie 97). Since they are unable to interact and live differently from what their passive role of patients predicts, they initially follow the hospital's rules, only to decide later to interrupt the treatment. Yet for those in higher social classes (Guizzetti 2008; Cobainsbaby; Gamberale; Vaniglia Orelli), this hierarchical social structure allows for new relational spaces with other anorexic/bulimic women.[6] Thanks to their higher cultural capital they are able to challenge the expertise of the medical staff. By opposing their knowledge to the medical system they reduce the power distance embedded in the hospital structure. They not only transgress their role as patients, but also continually reinterpret their hospital room, for example by furnishing it with personal knick-knacks or by inventing alternative leisure activities to those proposed and imposed by the hospital (Guizzetti, Cobainsbaby). Life in the hospital and the center for eating disorders produces ambivalent feelings. Initially, women feel protected from the external world while struggling to preserve their personal identity: "I also gave an identity to my refuge, by hanging my name tag on the door outside" (Guizzetti 35). In a second phase they invest their time and energy in the attempt to change the social and relational spaces here embodied. In this way, they first rediscover the chance to use their own capabilities with and for others and then, through others, the pleasure of gazing at, touching, and listening to something/someone outside themselves. In the last phase of their hospital stay they perceive the physical, social, and relational space of the center for eating disorders as too limiting and desire to return to the external world.

Conclusion

The main aim of this chapter was to understand how anorexic and bulimic women feel and experience their illness from a spatial-sociological perspective. Thus, unlike a psychoanalytic reading of anorexia, my interest was not in identifying the causes of anorexia, but in understanding how anorexia shapes the relationship between the body and space of anorexic women. From this viewpoint, social relationships are materially and discursively embodied in social and symbolic spaces. Also, while feminist literature analyzes anorexia by focusing on the interplay between body, space, and practices, I strayed from this framework on two pivotal points. First, according to feminist scholars, anorexia and bulimia result from the incorporation of patriarchal culture. However, even if we recognize that patriarchy (especially in the Catholic culture of Italy) still plays a relevant role in defining our social environment, this recognition should not obscure the other ways social and spatial processes interact with each other in (re)producing and transforming anorexic and bulimic behaviors and practices. The social and cultural norms embodied in the institutionalized spaces of the centers for eating disorders (or hospitals) are a good example of their influence in changing the anorexic or bulimic attitude, according to their cultural capital. Second, most feminist scholars to date have considered the process of becoming anorexic as driven by an intentional act. Following Darmon, I instead consider it as resulting from the consolidation of anorexic practices in an anorexic habitus and ethos as described in the autobiographies of anorexic/bulimic women.

Indeed, if we focus on the ways these women experience, perceive, categorize, and create boundaries between the mind and body, as well as between internal and external worlds during the "anorexic deviant career of conversion" (Darmon, "The Fifth Element" 718), it is clear how the initially intentional act of going on a diet as a means of self-control progressively leads to an increasing sense of symbolic and social disorientation, and ultimately to an escape from the spaces of everyday life leading to hospitalization (in twenty cases). However social and cultural differences among anorexic women modify the way they actualize their deviant career as anorexic/bulimic. During their anorexic careers, women of the lower middle class feel a greater sense of failure, which results in a more existentialist way of living in spaces and perceiving their bodies. The elevated level of family conflict and the persistence of a strong patriarchal culture counters their desire to realize themselves at school or in professional fields. As a consequence, the occurrence and persistence of anorexia/bulimia not only reinforces conflicts within the family but also the feeling of having no place, hence the only solution seems to starve themselves.

Notes

1 As psychoanalytic research underlines, anorexics and bulimics present similar behaviors, even though their relationship with food is quite different. In many of the cited narratives anorexics become bulimics; in those cases I will only use the term "anorexia" to indicate both.
2 The concept of habitus is taken from Bourdieu.
3 This aspect has been observed for all of the autobiographies, independent of their authors' sociocultural status.
4 The expressions "wicked viper" and "cancer of the soul" are used by Catholic authors.
5 This applies to all the authors, independent of their social position. What differs, however, is the length of this condition.
6 Thus the first circumstance concerns mostly the authors of the second group of autobiographies, whereas the second circumstance concerns the authors of the first and third groups.

Works Cited

Primary Literature

Arachi, Alessandra. *Briciole. Storia di un'anoressia*. Milan: Feltrinelli, 1994.

Artemisia. *Il cancro dell'anima: Diario di un'anoressia*. Rome: Intento, 2014.

Bandoli, Laura. *Questa non sono io: Anoressia e bulimia. Un'esperienza per capire*. Trento: Curcu & Genovese, 2008.

Boero, Michela. *Briciole di me*. Novate Milanese: Fabbrica dei segni, 2017.

Brunello, Clara. *Viva di nuovo: Come sono guarita dall'anoressia*. Milan: Edizioni Paoline, 2012.

Bruni, Aurora. *Mangia che ti passa: Diario di una ragazza in lotta contro l'anoressia*. Verona: Sansovino Press, 2000.

Cobainsbaby. *Il peso della felicità: I miei sedici anni tra anoressia e bulimia*. Milan: Mondadori, 2017.

De Clercq, Fabiola. *Tutto il pane del mondo: Cronaca di una vita tra anoressia e bulimia*. Florence: Sansoni, 1990.

Gamberale, Chiara. *Una vita sottile*. Venice: Marsilio, 2012.

Gardino, Daniela. *Al di là delle apparenze: Viaggio nell'anoressia*. Ravenna: SBC edizioni, 2008.

Grazioli, Erica. *Cioccolato e Cannella ... io e l'anoressia*. Milan: Selecta, 2017.

Guizzetti, Giuditta. *Il cucchiaio è una culla: Diario della battaglia di Yuyu contro l'anoressia*. Rome: Aliberti, 2008.

La Bella, Palma. *La farfalla dalle ali legate: Diario della mia anoressia*. Rome: Edizioni Magi, 2015.

Longo, Stefania. *Taglia trentotto: Bulimia, amore e rabbia*. Rome: Edizioni Memori, 2010.

Marzano, Michela. *Volevo essere una farfalle: Come l'anoressia mi ha insegnato a vivere*. Milan: Mondadori, 2011.

Miglietta, Anna. *Luce. Come l'anoressia mi ha seduta nel buio*. Acqui Terme: Editrice Impressioni grafiche, 2017.

Pasquadibisceglie, Nunzia. *Il vuoto dentro: L'esperienza dell'anoressia*. Tricase: Youcanprint, 2014.

Sabbadini, Stefania. *Trenta chili*. Rome: Nutrimenti, 2006.

Strappafelci, Maria Vittoria. *Il digiuno dell'anima: Una storia di anoressia*. Patti: Kimerik, 2016.

Tangheri, Nicoletta. *Il rumore dei miei passi: Una storia vera di anoressia*. Due Santi di Marino: Infinito, 2007.

Vaniglia Orelli, Ursula. *Mela Amara*, Rome: Iris, 2014.

Secondary Literature

Alpert, Augusta. "Reversibility of Pathological Fixations Associated with Maternal Deprivation in Infancy." *The Psychoanalytic Study of the Child* 14(1959): 169–185.

Boero, Natalie and C.J. Pascoe. "Pro-Anorexia Communities and Online Interaction: Bringing the Pro-ana Body Online." *Body and Society* 18. 2(2012): 27–57.

Bourdieu, Pierre. *Distinction: A Social Critique of the Judgement of Taste*. Cambridge: Harvard UP, 1979.

Bourdieu, Pierre. "The Forms of Capital." *Handbook of Theory and Research for the Sociology of Education*. Ed. J. Richardson. New York: Greenwood, 1986. 241–258.

Bourdieu, Pierre. *Outline of a Theory of Practice*. Cambridge: Cambridge UP, 1972.

Bray, Abigail and Claire Colebrook. "The Haunted Flesh: Corporeal Feminism and the Politics of (Dis)embodiment." *Signs* 24. 1(1998): 35–67.

Bruch, Hilde. "Hunger and Instinct." *Journal of Nervous and Mental Disease* 149. 2(1969): 91–114.

Butler, Judith. "Performative Acts and Gender Constitution: An Essay in Phenomenology and Feminist Theory." *Theatre Journal* 40. 4(1998): 519–531.

Caruana, Louis. "Somatic Semantics: Anorexia and the Nature of Meaning." *Anorexia Nervosa: A Multidisciplinary Approach: From Biology to Philosophy*. Ed. Antonio Mancini, Silvia Daini and Louis Caruana. New York: Nova Science Publishers, 2010. 173–186.

Crisp, Arthur H. *Anorexia Nervosa: Let me Be*. London: Academic Press, 1980.

Crisp, Arthur H. "Psychological Aspect of Breast Feeding with Particular Reference to Anorexia Nervosa." *British Journal of Medical Psychology* 42(1969): 119–132.

Darmon, Muriel. *Devenir anorexique: Une approche sociologique*. Paris: Editions la Decouverte, 2003.

Darmon, Muriel. "The Fifth Element: Social Class and the Sociology of Anorexia." *Sociology* 43. 4(2009): 717–733.

Debord, Guy. *La société du spectacle*. Paris: Buchet/Chastel, 1967.

Di Viggiano, Pasquale Luigi and Rossella Bufano. *Donna e società: Partecipazione democratica e cittadinanza digitale*. Trento: Tangram, 2013.

Duncan, Nancy, ed. *BodySpace: Destabilizing Geographies of Gender and Sexuality*. London: Routledge, 1996.

Garrett, Catherine J. "Recovery from Anorexia Nervosa: A Durkheimian Interpretation." *Social Science and Medicine* 43. 10(1996): 1489–1506.

Goffman, Erving. *Asylums: Essays on the Social Situation of Mental Patients and other Inmates*. New York: Random House, 1961.

Goode, Erich. *Deviant Behavior*. Englewood Cliffs: Prentice-Hall, 1978.

Grazian, David. "Urban Nightlife, Social Capital and the Public Life of Cities." *Sociological Forum* 24. 4(2009): 908–917.

Grosz, Elizabeth A. *Space, Time and Perversion: Essays on the Politics of Bodies.* London: Routledge, 2005.

Grüning, Barbara and René Tuma. "Space, Interaction and Communication: Sociology in Dialogue with Spatial Studies: An Introduction." *Sociologica* 2(2017): 1–16.

Hochschild, Arlie. "Emotion Work, Feeling Rules, and Social Structure." *American Journal of Sociology* 85. 3(1979): 551–575.

Irigaray, Luce. *Elemental Passions.* London: Athlone Press, 1992.

Knoblauch, Hubert and Löw, Martina. "On the Spatial Refiguration of the Social World." *Sociologica* 2(2017): 1–27.

Löw, Martina. "The Constitution of Space: The Structuration of Spaces through the Simultaneity of Effect and Perception." *European Journal of Social Theory* 11. 1(2008): 25–49.

Löw, Martina. *Raumsoziologie.* Frankfurt/M: Suhrkamp, 2001.

MacSween, Morag. *Anorexic Body: A Feminist and Sociological Perspective on Anorexia Nervosa.* London: Routledge, 1989.

Maione, Valeria. *Insiemesipuò: Gli stati generali delle Donne nelle regioni italiane.* Milan: Angeli, 2016.

Malagoli Togliatti, Marisa. "Disagio adolescenziale e strutture famigliari deboli." *Psicologia clinica dello sviluppo* 1(1998): 73–97.

Malson, Helen. *The Thin Woman: Feminism, Post-Structuralism and the Social Psychology of Anorexia Nervosa.* London: Routledge, 1998.

Massey, Doreen. *For Space.* London: Sage, 2005.

Massey, Doreen. *Space, Place and Gender.* Minneapolis: U of Minnesota P, 1994.

McRobbie, Angela. *The Aftermath of Feminism: Gender, Culture and Social Change.* Thousand Oaks: Sage, 2008.

Mead, Georg Herbert. *Minds, Self and Society.* Chicago: U of Chicago P, 1934.

Minuchin, Salvador, Bernice Rosman, and Lester Baker. *Psychosomatic Families: Anorexia Nervosa in Context.* Cambridge: Harvard UP, 1978.

Moss, Pamela and Isabel Dyck. *Women, Body, Illness: Space and Identity in the Everyday Lives of Women with Chronic Illness.* Lanham: Rowman and Littlefield Publishers, 2003.

O'Connor, Richard A. and Penny Van Esterik. "De-Medicalizing Anorexia: A New Cultural Brokering." *Anthropology Today* 24. 5(2008): 6–9.

Orbach, Susie. "Accepting the Symptom: A Feminist Psychoanalytic Treatment of Anorexia Nervosa." *Handbook of Psychotherapy for Anorexia Nervosa and Bulimia.* Ed. D. Garner and P. Garfinkel. New York: Guilford, 1985. 83–106.

Orbach, Susie. *Hunger Strike: The Anorexic's Struggle as a Metaphor for our Age.* New York: Norton, 1986.

Ostuzzi, Roberto and Gian Luigi Luxardi. "Le metafore della bulimia." *Salute e società* 3(2009): 123–141.

Parr, Hester and Ruth Butler. "New Geographies of Illness, Impairment and Disability." *Mind and Body Spaces.* Ed. R. Butler and H. Parr. London: Routledge, 1999. 1–24.

Puwar, Nirmal. *Space Invaders: Race, Gender and Bodies Out of Place.* Oxford: Berg, 2004.

Recalcati, Massimo. *L'uomo senza inconscio.* Milan: Cortina, 2010.

Rich, Emma. "Anorexic (Dis)connection: Managing Anorexia as an Illness and an Identity." *Sociology of Health and Illness* 28. 3(2006): 284–305.

Robson, Kathryn. "Voicing Abjection: Narratives of Anorexia in Contemporary French Women's (Life-)Writing." *L'Esprit Créateur* 56. 2(2016): 108–120.

Selvini Palazzoli, Mara. *Self-Starvation*. New York: Jason Aronson, 1963.

Silva, Elizabeth B. "Habitus: Beyond Sociology." *The Sociological Review* 64(2016): 73–92.

Slade, Roger. *The Anorexia Nervosa Reference Book: Direct and Clear Answers to Everyone's Questions*. New York: Harper and Rowe, 1984.

Sperling, Melitta. "The Role of the Mother in Psychosomatic Disorders in Children." *Psychosomatic Medicine* 11(1949): 377–385.

Turner, Bryan S. *Regulating Bodies: Essays in Medical Sociology*. London: Routledge, 1992.

Vander Ven, Thomas and Marikay Vander Ven. "Exploring Patterns of Mother-Blaming in Anorexia Scholarship: A Study in the Sociology of Knowledge." *Human Studies* 26 (2003): 97–119.

Wacquant, Loïc. "Habitus as Topic and Tool: Reflections on Becoming a Prizefighter." *Qualitative Research in Psychology* 8(2011): 81–92.

Warin, Megan. *Abject Relations: Everyday Worlds of Anorexia*. New Brunswick: Rutgers UP, 2010.

Part II

Invasive Influences and Corporeal Integrity

7 Unseen Enemies

Neisseria, Desire, and Bodily Discourse

Lisa M. DeTora

Introduction

In her TEDx Orange talk, "Living Beyond Limits" (2011), Amy Purdy, a survivor of meningococcal septicemia who would go on to be a paralympian snowboarder and *Dancing with the Stars* runner-up, begins by asking a question: how each member of her audience would want their own story to go. When Purdy begins her own uplifting personal narrative, she implies that she, herself, is the author of her words, that she is telling the audience how she wants her story to go. And it seems that she is, except where she borrows from common public health and medical narratives to describe the devastating consequences of meningococcal disease, which took her legs below the knees, her spleen, her kidneys, and the hearing in her left ear. In fact, in less than a day, Purdy's body had transitioned from the excellent fitness necessary for her as professional snowboarder to the brink of death. She initially believed she had "the flu," but "less than 24 hours later," she was "in the hospital, on life support, with a less than 2% chance of living." It took days before she was "diagnosed with 'bacterial meningitis,' a vaccine-preventable blood infection" (TEDx). Her narrative walks listeners through her tale, adding layers to Purdy's body of experience as well as the experience of her body. Ultimately, the narrative offers its readers the image of a superpositional meningococcal body: one that coalesces into a new type of existence as each new element comes into play. Thus, Purdy occupies not one, but many bodily states in the course of her narrative, and, in fact, ultimately comes to occupy all of them at once.

This chapter theorizes the possibility for a meningococcal body as a site of multiple conformations and experiences and as a possible site of identity formation. The meningococcal body dovetails with Donna Haraway's notion of the cyborg as a figure for humanity imbricated with machine, a possibility for a type of identity that transcends older modes of gender identification. Haraway is an important cultural precursor to current theories of posthumanity, which problematize the relationship of human bodies not only with technology but also with the microbiological world. Thus, the meningococcal body exposes the means by which combination with and habitation by other bodies, like those of bacteria, creates a space for myriad superpositional engagements. Ultimately, the meningococcal body stands in for the ecological relationship between the human body and the creatures that inhabit it. The meningococcal body is an entity that depends on the intervention of the foreign bodies of bacteria.

The material assembled below suggests that the simultaneous mobilization of human and microbiological desire, a model borrowed from visual semiotics, can create new embodied states. These embodied states, like Haraway's cyborgs or the many affordances of posthuman theories of pathological states, trouble existing constructions of the body. But, further than this, the superpositions required to create and understand the meningococcal body offer a vantage point for what might be termed a quantum understanding of embodiment: an understanding that holds many nascent possibilities and conceptual frames in tension at once.

Superpositional Bodies and Conceptual Frames

A "quantum" understanding of embodiment involves an understanding of quantum states, or the ability of the denizens of the quantum world, or subatomic particles, to occupy more than one place, position, value, or "state" at once. In quantum physics, different subatomic systems can occupy multiple quantum states simultaneously, creating new quantum states. This "layering" of quantum states and the new quantum states that such layering creates occur through "superposition." Also important to the current discussion, observation itself can alter an established quantum state, that is, the exact location and value of a specific particle, because of the differences in scale between the human observer and the subatomic particle. In other words, human observation can fix quantum states, which until then remained unclear. In positing the existence of a meningococcal body, superposition serves as a model for any system or entity occupying multiple states at the same time. The idea that observation changes superpositional states can contribute to this model. Thus, superposition can be used to understand the cultural and other means of figuring embodiment. Such an understanding will necessitate specific powers of perception and an intellectual means of framing them.

I use the idea of framing following Lakoff and Johnson's theoretical treatment of cognitive framing through the use of metaphor in *Metaphors We Live By*. These cognitive psychologists recognize that ideas and things lack meaning unless some conceptual frame exists to house them. In the setting of infection, a critical frame is what Michel Foucault referred to as a "medical gaze" in *The Birth of the Clinic: An Archaeology of Medical Perception*. For Foucault, the medical gaze is a function of perception as linked to language, which he describes as "paradoxical" (108) as well as simultaneous. The gaze of a physician or researcher can see past the specific experience of a patient to the activities of microbes or an underlying disease, a significant intellectual development in the field of medicine. The medical gaze also creates language capable of translating or conveying these perceptions to others: researchers, patients, colleagues.

However, as with most theoretical models, the necessary connection of language and spectacles or bodies in the Foucauldian construction of a medical gaze, has its limits. A key example, and an essential frame for feminist conceptions of the body, is the "domain of unthinkable, abject, unliveable bodies" (xi) that Judith Butler describes as "culturally unintelligible" in *Bodies that Matter: On the Discursive Limits of Sex*. For Butler, these bodies escape the boundaries of knowledge, but not experience, and therefore may be especially susceptible to manifestations of power that problematize performances of identity and gender. Further, because gender performance cannot be picked up and set down at will, the manifestation of the inevitable consequences of power relations on bodies creates gender, hence identity. Given that all cultural ideas about the body, especially the human body, are essentially gendered, the conditions for defining the self or the subject require certain performances. Such performances may continue to defy the usual bounds of gender once they enter posthuman discourses of gender.

Purdy navigates the horrific—the abject or unlivable—elements of her story in part by describing the ways she can now alter her legs and feet at will using various technologies. Thus, for Purdy, her experience of meningococcal disease is the dividing line between the old Amy and a new Amy, creating another superpositional state for her audience, which is the result of a near-fatal infection that links her old and new selves. The new Amy also builds her narrative around a public health story, which incorporates different bodily states and medical terminologies intended to motivate governments and individuals to mandate, fund, and receive vaccines. Thus, Purdy's personal narrative holds multiple discourses—personal, medical, public, popular—in tension, setting the stage for a specific metaphoric construction of the meningococcal body.

Superposition as Inspiration

All bodies matter, of course, but Purdy's can be said to matter more than most because of its cultural intelligibility in several different social and intellectual discourses. Purdy may be said to matter even more because of her ability to reconfigure, and transition, her body by the simple act of changing her feet, an act that she represents as a common-sense way of managing performance in the face of physical limitation. In the public media and her book, *On My Own Two Feet* (2014), Purdy resembles the heroine of a Horatio Alger narrative, overcoming a disfiguring and potentially disabling illness only to undertake a series of physically and emotionally challenging occupations, inspiring millions by her courage and resilience in the face of what would be crippling adversity for most people.

The dominant narrative about Purdy, here taken from the PBS *Medal Quest* web site, goes like this:

> at 19, she [Purdy] contracted a particularly virulent form of bacterial meningitis. She went into septic shock, which led to double amputation below the knees and the loss of her spleen and a kidney. Doctors gave her a 2% chance of survival.

Beating the odds, she survived, and her indomitable spirit helped her
back to the [snowboarding] slopes.

Within this narrative, Purdy transitions between multiple dichotomous identities:
able/disabled, healthy/ill, victim/victor, snowboarder/double amputee; to name
only a few. She effects these transitions through the power of an "indomitable
spirit." As Purdy explains in "Living Beyond Limits," just as she realized her
dream to be a snowboarder and physical therapist, she contracted invasive
meningococcal meningitis and septicemia. Yet, even though Purdy had only "a
2% chance" to live, a detail included even in sound bite descriptions, she decided
not only to live, but to expand her ambitions. These transitions, on examination,
coalesce into a superpositional identity, at once disabled and exceptional,
simultaneously enacting many elements.

In public, Purdy glows with charisma and confidence, insisting that meningococcal disease impacted her self-concept without transforming her into a
disease victim. Purdy took a bronze medal in snowboarding in the 2014 Paralympic games, a sport she introduced to the games. Later that year, she took
second place on *Dancing with the Stars*, behind Olympic gold medalist Meryl
Davis. More significantly for the purposes of this chapter, Purdy continues her
bodily transitions—superpositioning herself physically as well as culturally—
every time she builds new legs or changes her feet. As she explains, once she
realized that she could now be as tall or nearly as short as she wanted and her
feet would never get cold, a whole new world of possibilities opened before her.
Purdy works with her altered body, channeling it to her ends, rather than suc-
cumbing to the limitations imposed by disease. This persona continues from her
TEDx talk through her Paralympic and *Dancing With the Stars* interviews and
even to a later diagnosis of rhabdomyolysis, a rare disease that denatures
skeletal protein and impacts kidney health (Enriquez).

Purdy's personal narratives, both those she constructs as well as the ones that
are framed about her, simultaneously incorporate and contravene generally
accepted narratives about meningococcal disease, which tend to emphasize
untoward consequences in order to encourage public health measures, such as
vaccination.

Defining the Meningococcal Body

In defining the meningococcal body it is important to understand *Neisseria
meningitidis*, the meningococcus (see Van de Beek and Van de Beek et al.). The
meningococcus is an obligate human parasite: it can live nowhere else except in
a human body. It most commonly dwells in the human nasopharynx, a space
shared with other species of microflora. A few of these microflora, like the
meningococcus, pneumococcus, and *Staphylococcus aureus*, can become deadly
pathogens. The meningococcus is unusual among potentially pathogenic, or
disease-causing, organisms because it has no other animal or environmental
reservoirs. It is unusual among members of its own genus, because most

obligate parasites tend not to cause disease in their hosts. The meningococcus is a human-specific organism that sometimes happens to kill.

In the popular imagination, the word "infection" implies an active disease, symptoms, illness, or sickness. However, as the meningococcus does not cause illness in its ideal state, medical discourses sometimes parse fine distinctions between colonization, asymptomatic carriage, and invasive infection. Nevertheless, the most common definition of "infection"—the introduction of a pathogen or potential pathogen into a body—seems to cover all these scenarios, from an organism happening to live in the body to an infectious disease. This, like Purdy's various states of selfhood, is an instance of a quantum bodily state: the ability for the body to be healthy and infected at once.

Most meningococcal infections fall into a category of asymptomatic carriage, which indicates that the nasopharynx is inhabited by the bacteria without any signs of disease. Usually, about 10 to 20% of the human population carries meningococci at any one time. Certain factors increase the odds of carriage, and some groups have more risk of acquiring the bacteria or contracting active disease. In adolescents and young adults, smoking or exposure to cigarette smoke, moving into a college dormitory or military quarters, and going to pubs or clubs, all increase opportunities to acquire *Neisseria*. But these are only odds. Nearly every human body can become a meningococcal body, that is, a body inhabited by the meningococcus, without experiencing lasting harm. The transition from unaffected person to carrier, from uninfected to infected, can begin and end without any signs or symptoms. These bodies remain, to all intents and purposes, healthy, and in fact, may be both healthy and infected. This circumstance is necessary for the continued survival of the meningococcus, which requires this superposition to survive.

To remain alive, the meningococcus also must evade the human complement system, a series of proteins that help the body's innate defenses against infection (Lucidarme et al.). Scientific papers tend to describe the meningococcus as developing strategies to evade the complement system, ensuring continued survival. If the meningococcus enters the human blood stream, a transition from benign to invasive infection, catastrophic results ensue, like those Purdy experienced. Yet invasive meningococcal disease, like every other aspect of meningococcal existence, is also superpositional, a constellation of frightening, sudden-onset illnesses that can kill or maim an otherwise healthy individual—usually an infant or a teenager—in mere hours, even with prompt medical treatment. The bacteria replicate rapidly in the bloodstream, shutting down essential bodily functions, causing a disfiguring bleeding rash, failed circulation, organ failure, and/or gangrene, literally disintegrating the body. Even if antibiotics are used to eradicate the bacteria, permanent disability, disfigurement, or death result. Ironically, the danger of invasive disease is equally serious for the meningococcus because it cannot live outside of a human host, and if the host dies, so do the bacteria. The very existence of the meningococcus, then, relies on the ability of the human body to simultaneously harbor and withstand it, sitting on the knife's edge between health and disease. Therefore, the medical narratives that surround this organism and the people affected by it, like Purdy's narrative, require a reader to hold seemingly disparate ideas in tension, superimposed on one another.

In this discussion, the human body serves only as a backdrop for various biological processes that take place on cellular or molecular scales. The impersonal nasopharyngeal space of this human body lacks subjectivity and agency, which instead are assigned to bacteria and cells, following the military paradigm of disease described by Susan Sontag. Sontag traces the "history of metaphorical thinking about the body" that "features catastrophe" (8). These military metaphors gained traction with the discovery of microbiological pathogens, an identifiable enemy, eventually coming to "infuse all aspects of the description of the medical situation" (9), casting disease as villain and patients as victims. In the militarized discourses of infection that Sontag examines, like the scientific discussion of the meningococcus, the human body is merely a backdrop to more interesting events, a geography to be colonized, conquered, or defended. In other words, medical discussions of the meningococcus construct it as being like other harmful cells, bent on destruction, creating yet another site of superposition, that of all possible bacteria and viruses bent on attacking the human body.

Yet meningococcal bodies matter more in both performative and cultural terms, than simple terrain. The meningococcal body does more than simply sit at a knife's edge of infected-yet-healthy, but rather superpositions myriad epistemological positions. Of note, by describing her own illness as vaccine preventable, Purdy, who contracted the disease years before a vaccine was available for the particular serogroup that caused her illness, stretches the truth. Her story functions as public health morality tale and post-hoc caution, designed to protect others rather than to reveal her past. It is a tale that shows how meningococcal disease ravages bodies, creating sudden transition from health not merely to illness but to scenes of abject horror.

Superposition as Performance

Purdy's narrative presents only one version of the meningococcal body. This body is not always gendered, especially when it falls away to become the backdrop for microbiological dramas. Like every other body transformed by infection, the meningococcal body shifts, but with a difference because its relationships to specific microflora and disease states are superpositioned, requiring the observer to consider multiple states of being at once. A further superposition, both for Purdy's story and a medical understanding of the disease, is the dominant public health narrative of meningococcal disease.

Purdy's account of her illness bears many of the hallmarks of public health narratives that describe the effects of invasive meningococcal infections on the bodies of patients. For example, 2015 student fact sheets about meningococcal disease distributed by the University of Buffalo present a list of early symptoms and cautions:

The early symptoms usually associated with meningococcal disease include fever, severe headache, stiff neck, rash, nausea, vomiting, and lethargy, and may resemble the flu. Because the disease progresses rapidly, often in as little as 12 hours, students are urged to seek medical care immediately if they experience two or more of these symptoms concurrently.

Similarly, a student fact sheet from the University of California at Merced states:

> Meningococcal disease is often misdiagnosed as something less serious, as the symptoms often resemble those of the flu. Symptoms may include sudden high fever, headache, stiff neck, nausea, vomiting and exhaustion. Some people also develop a rash. Since symptoms progress quickly, it is very important that medical attention is sought immediately.

Both of these fact sheets, like more recent documents at SUNY Oswego or Marquette University, emphasize the dangers of thinking that any sudden illness is the flu, as Purdy did at the time, and also the rapid progression of disease from mild flulike symptoms to life-threatening illness. Until meningococcal disease is successfully diagnosed by the operation of the medical gaze, these bodies may, in fact, suffer from only an ordinary illness; however, these cautions superposition the possibility for sudden, devastating illness on what most likely are ordinary aches and pains, creating an essential site of uncertainty.

The cautions on these fact sheets are joined, in Purdy's narrative, with the term vaccine-preventable to describe her blood infection (or septicemia). The use of such language is unsurprising given her position as a spokesperson for Pfizer, a maker of meningococcal vaccines. The discourse of vaccine prevention Purdy mobilizes most often centers not on the people being protected, but on the bacteria that cause disease. Purdy's story, then, can be seen to participate in public health discourses that present considerations of the body on microbiological and whole human scales, toggling between horrifying images of life support and missing limbs to highly impersonal images of microbiological activities occurring against the backdrop of a depersonalized human body made possible by Foucault's medical gaze. These discursive transitions between bodily representations inform literal transitions in what I term the meningococcal body, creating a site of multiple superpositions.

Superposition as Anxiety

Purdy's narrative is only one possible story of the meningococcal body: a story of triumph and overcoming obstacles. The fact sheets quoted above, unlike Purdy's TEDx talk, provide a truncated narrative—their aim is to intervene before disease occurs. If one continued the cautions in these college information sheets, a typical meningococcal disease narrative might go like this:

An otherwise healthy person, usually an infant or a young man or woman just starting a new phase in life (college, boarding school, the military) begins to feel mildly unwell. The early symptoms are not particularly concerning. In fact, it seems like a cold or perhaps a case of the flu. However, something is just not right, and parents or the young person seek medical attention.

The lucky ones will find medical practitioners who recognize the early signs of bacterial meningitis or septicemia, but some of these ill persons will arrive at medical centers with less experience. Within a matter of hours, all of these children or young adults will become dangerously ill. Some will die.

Even when an appropriate antibiotic is administered in time to save a life, about 20% of these patients will experience some type of serious side effect. Meningitis can cause brain and other neurological damage, resulting in emotional and cognitive problems or deficits. For those who develop septicemia, or blood poisoning, gangrene can set into the extremities, causing loss of fingers, toes, or whole limbs. Organs such as the kidney or spleen can suffer irreparable damage. Hearing can be affected, and severe scarring may result if the injuries heal. Scar tissue can be disfiguring, but more seriously, it can impair muscular function and induce chronic pain. These effects last a lifetime, causing largely untold suffering and creating persistent societal and health resource burdens.

In this telling of meningococcal disease, the undesired outcomes are disability, disfigurement, impairment, or death. Absent from this understanding of the disease is Purdy's inspirational message, her ability to create her own feet, to transform herself and her life at will. Purdy herself layers these images, but the typical narrative does not; it remains stabilized in the space of disability.

Ashley Lee, a young woman who contracted meningococcal meningitis in 2005, exemplifies these more typical narratives. As NBC reporter Melissa Dahl writes, "After multiple surgeries and the amputation of a foot and three fingers … [Ashley] strives each day to cope with her new reality." Ashley struggles daily with cosmetic issues caused by scars as well as chronic pain in her amputated limb. She depends on pain medication, which is a troublesome requirement in the midst of the opioid addiction epidemic, to function on a daily basis. The worst part of Ashley's story is that she tried to get vaccinated just weeks before she became ill, but the doctor's office had run out of doses.

In Ashley's narrative, the best outcomes or even a return to normal life, are absent in part because public health rhetoric is intended to spur action like the introduction of a vaccine, improved early detection in emergency rooms, better antibiotic protocols, or even education for pediatricians and school administrators. Ashley illustrates the consequences of leaving a needed vaccine until later, including the unintended emotional toll of "never letting my guard down," even around her closest friends, who insist that she is just the same as ever, even if she can no longer pump her own gas with a disfigured hand. The bodies of the survivors here transition from health to deathly illness to permanent disability and deficit, leaving their old selves behind. Ashley's body, unlike Purdy's, is a cautionary tale, intended to warn the still healthy that it is not too late to prevent disease. These narratives mobilize a utilitarian medical ethics, victimizing certain survivors in order to save others. Ashley, unlike Purdy, does not proudly sport a series of unique and creative prosthetics that expand her possibilities.

Significantly, the superposition in Ashley's story is intended to incorporate the listener. Rather than creating a series of empowering personal identifications, like Purdy's first-person narrative, news coverage of Ashley's story imparts a sense of doom. Ashley's choices were over the instant she was denied a dose of meningococcal vaccine; perhaps, had she been more persistent, she would not have lost her foot and fingers, would not be lying to her friends, would be able to pump gas. Here, meningococcal disease clearly demarcates not a boundary between two different types of personal fulfillment and empowerment, but the dividing line between normal health and the type of abjection Butler describes as culturally unintelligible. Ashley cannot frame her experience in language, and therefore hides her feelings and her pain in order to take a place in society. Ashley's story invites the listener to superposition her experiences onto theirs, not to embrace them, but to reject an unlivable reality by getting vaccinated.

Bodily Integrity

One of the most frightening aspects of meningococcal disease is the rapid deterioration of the body, the transition from a healthy person to something else. The image of this type of failing, even disintegrating, body, simultaneously fascinates—as in a popular preoccupation with zombies—and haunts—as with H5N1 influenza or ebola—the public imagination. Daniel Dinello argues that the cultural importance of "horrific images of mutilated bodies and corrupted flesh" (246) increased with the end of the Cold War and the cessation of the persistent nuclear threat that held the superpowers in check. I suggest that these posthuman visions provide another site of superposition, and a cultural one, in which meningococcal disease operates.

In his discussion of turn of the twenty-first century science fiction films like *28 Days Later* (2002) and more verisimilitudinous movies like *Outbreak* (1995), Dinello reads against a larger narrative of infectious disease anxiety, including ebola, the 1999 outbreak of West Nile Virus in the United States, or the threat of H5N1 influenza. These microbiological threats to humanity supplanted nuclear Armageddon as the most feared possible cause of the collapse of civilization, infecting the public imagination. Freed from the possibility that the United States and the former Soviet Union would decimate the world's population with nuclear warheads, popular culture took up the potential for plagues to wreak havoc, creating a different, but no less disturbing, apocalyptic vision. As Dinello explains, cultural productions retained the basic nuclear

Armageddon narrative, slotting in disease for the communist aggressor, and creating a need for fictions to address or sublimate the "mutilated bodies and corrupted flesh" (246) of the infected and make way for what he terms post-humanity. Dinello notes that science fiction traces the proliferation of creatures like zombies and vampires to infectious agents, suggesting that a transition from humanity to posthumanity, an amalgam of biological and technological humanity, is the only possible future. Dinello also discovers that even the technology that might promise salvation in a cyborg future is not immune to microbiological contamination, as the Coen Brothers show in *The Matrix* franchise. Cyborgs and machines, in fact, remain susceptible to viral infection, thus negating the promise of immortality through machines.

The circular narrative of infectious Armageddon remains important in such discussions because it informs scientific discourses as well as fictional ones. As Robert Webster and Elizabeth Walker note in an *American Scientist* essay, the story of the 1918 H1N1 pandemic, or the putative H5N1 pandemic is "like a cheesy Hollywood horror flick" (122), the precise type of film Dinello discusses in his book. Webster and Walker cast disease as a "shape-shifting killer" (123) that nimbly outmaneuvers medical and scientific intervention, leaving millions dead. Although these authors describe this plot as a sophomoric idea for a movie script, they acknowledge that it captures the bill when describing the trajectory of the 1918 Spanish influenza. In 1918, troop movements from the Great War helped spread the especially virulent H1N1 flu strain across the globe.

Meningococcal disease may be less common than influenza, but its history is also characterized by military interventions and horrific images, creating an additional site for cultural and historical superposition. The septicemic form of the disease was first described in 1805 by Gaspard Vissieux, but the meningo-coccus itself was not discovered until decades later, in 1887. The initial description of the disease in the absence of its cause was made possible by characteristic clinical features that differentiated it from other diseases that traveled, along with troops, across war-riddled areas. Meningococcal disease, unlike other similar fevers, caused rapid progression and decline, leading to death in more than 80% of patients within the first two days of the initial symptoms. The distinctive features of the diseases were disfiguring, bleeding, impacting bodily integrity. Survivors were often left deaf and/or blind. Of interest, this literal military overlap with the medical history of the meningo-coccus creates a further site for theoretical superpositioning, tying the meta-phoric language of evasion and invasion with past material discourses of infection and disease.

Unseen Enemies

This chapter began with the idea of superposition and continues to illustrate how layering can incorporate bodies (bacteria/human), experiences (abject/empowered), histories (military/personal), and discourses (public health/science fiction). A common thread in these discourses is the meningococcal body, the once and future habitation of a specific bacteria that must have a human host. This model of the body violates dominant social narratives even as it reinforces them. As sociologist of medicine Deborah Lupton explains, people in developed nations expect continuously good health at minimal cost with little to no inconvenience. What Lupton termed the "imperative of health" draws on Foucault and contributes to a series of paradoxical views of medicine as highly suspect and incredibly prestigious. Yet this paradox can extend beyond developed countries into the regions most strongly affected by meningococcal disease like sub-Saharan Africa, superpositioning persons of all races, genders, and economic and social circumstances. By mirroring science fiction horrors as well as stories of personal empowerment, meningococcal narratives reside not only on the knife's edge between illness and health but also the dividing line between truth and fiction. By seeing the meningococcal body as a means of unifying all people, not merely through the technologically-oriented model of posthumanity that informs Haraway's cyborg but also through the narrative conventions that Dinello examines, this superpositional figure has the potential to problematize race and gender not only in the developed world but also globally.

Works Cited

Boyle, Danny, dir. *28 Days Later*. United States: 20th Century Fox Home Entertainment, 2003.

Butler, Judith. *Bodies that Matter: On the Discursive Limits of Sex*. New York: Routledge, 1993.

Dahl, Melissa. "Killer at College: Meningitis Threatens Students." *NBC News*. 2007. www.nbcnews.com/id/20519953/ns/health-infectious_diseases/t/killer-college-meningit is-threatens-students/#.VM5iecZ4aDo.

Dancing with the Stars. Season Nineteen. ABC.

Dinello, Daniel. *Technophobia: Science Fiction Visions of Posthuman Technology*. Austin: U of Texas P, 1995.

Enriquez, Justin. "'This Condition Is So Scary': Paralympic Snowboarder and DWTS Alum Amy Purdy Rushed to ER and Diagnosed with Rhabdomyolysis." *Daily Mail* 27 October 2016.

Foucault, Michel. *The Birth of the Clinic: An Archaeology of Medical Perception*. Trans. A.M. Sheridan Smith. New York: Vintage, 1994.

Haraway, Donna. "A Cyborg Manifesto: Science, Technology, and Socialist-Feminism in the Late Twentieth Century." *Simians, Cyborgs and Women: The Reinvention of Nature*. New York: Routledge, 1991. 149–181.

Lakoff, George and Mark Johnson. *Metaphors We Live by*. Chicago, IL: U of Chicago P, 2003.

Lucidarme, Jay, Lionel Tan, Rachel M. Exley, Jamie Findlow, Ray Borrow, and Christoph M. Tang. "Characterization of *Neisseria meningitidis* Isolates That Do Not Express the Virulence Factor and Vaccine Antigen Factor H Binding Protein." *Clinical Vaccine Immunology* 18. 6(2011): 1002–1014.

Lupton, Deborah. *Medicine as Culture: Illness, Disease and the Body*. New York: Sage, 2012.

Marquette University. "Meningococcal Disease." www.marquette.edu/medical-clinic/resources-meningococcal.shtml.

PBS. "Amy Purdy." *Medal Quest: American Athletes and the Paralympic Games*. www.pbs.org/wgbh/medal-quest/athletes/detail/amy-purdy/.

Peterson, Wolfgang, dir. *Outbreak*. United States: Warner Bros, 1997.

Purdy, Amy. "Living Beyond Limits." *TEDx Orange Coast*. May 2011. Available at: www.ted.com/talks/amy_purdy_living_beyond_limits.

Purdy, Amy. *On My Own Two Feet: From Losing My Legs to Learning the Dance of Life*. New York: Harper Collins, 2014.

Sontag, Susan. *Illness as Metaphor and AIDS and Its Metaphors*. New York: Doubleday, 1990.

SUNY Oswego. Walker Health Center. "Meningococcal Disease Information." www.oswego.edu/walker-health-center/meningococcal-disease-information.

University of Buffalo. "Fact Sheet." 2015.

University of California at Merced. "Fact Sheet." 2015.

Van de Beek, Diederik. "Advances in Treatment of Bacterial Meningitis." *Lancet* 380. 9854(2012): 1693–1702.

Van de Beek, Diederik, Jan de Gans, Lodewijk Spanjaard, Martijn Weisfelt, Johannes B. Reitsma, and Marinus Vermeulen. "Clinical Features and Prognostic Factors in Adults with Bacterial Meningitis." *New England Journal of Medicine* 351(2004): 1849–1859.

Wachowski, Andy, and Larry Wachowski, dir. *The Matrix*. Burbank, CA: Warner Home Video, 1999.

Webster, Robert G, and Elizabeth Jane Walker. "Influenza: The World is Teetering on the Edge of a Pandemic that Could Kill a Large Fraction of the Human Population." *American Scientist* 91. 2(2003): 122–129.

8 The Human Papillomavirus Vaccination

Gendering the Rhetorics of Immunization in Public Health Discourses

Jennifer A. Malkowski

Gender is often invoked to sell health products and behaviors in various public and professional discourses. Susan Bordo speaks to the intersections of patriarchal culture and capitalist ideologies in *Unbearable Weight: Feminism, Western Culture and the Body* (2004). By making sense of anorexia as a mediated cultural, social, and medical phenomenon, Bordo identifies important evidence of the intolerable pressures facing American women. Ultimately, she argues, the consequences of the tension between patriarchy and consumer behavior fall disproportionately on the shoulders of American women. Yet weight loss is not the only site of this "unbearable weight." The current chapter examines how specific rhetorical practices—particularly the discourse of human papillomavirus (HPV) vaccines—in health and medicine disproportionately impact women's lives by equating certain health conditions with biological sex. Cervical cancer is only one of many potential outcomes of HPV, yet across media and messages the two have been treated as somewhat synonymous. This inaccuracy prohibits men from fully entering the conversation and disproportionately shifts the burden of responsibility for the management of this particular condition to women.

A large body of literature challenges the conflation of biological or anatomical factors and gender (Lorber), yet an ill-defined appeal to biology continues to be used as a gender sense-making device across many health settings and issues. In her book *The Sociology of Gender*, Amy Wharton examines the difference between sex and gender, the intersection of gender and culture, and theories of how we become gendered. For Wharton, "gender is as much of a process as a fixed state"; it "is not simply a characteristic of individuals, but occurs at all levels of the social structure" and "is one critical dimension upon which social resources are distributed" (9). She emphasizes that "gender involves the creation of both differences *and* inequalities" (8). In line with Wharton, Candace West and Don H. Zimmerman note that "when we view gender as an accomplishment, an achieved property of situated conduct, our attention shifts from matters internal to the individual and focuses on interactional and, ultimately, institutional arenas" (126). For the practices of health and medicine, in particular, gender gets used as "a powerful ideological device, which produces, reproduces, and legitimates choices and limits that are predicated on sex category" (147). Even though sophisticated modes of inquiry identify limits to anatomical markers of sex, less sophisticated discourses continue to appeal to anatomical determinism in direct opposition to the view that gender is socially constructed. Bordo's exploration of the female body as it relates to power and control is only one analysis that suggests that the biological–social distinction of gender remains contested.

Commonly framed in terms of the "public good" and therefore presumably gender-neutral, vaccination may be an ironic location for gendered discourse. Yet that changed in the current century with the introduction of human papillomavirus (HPV) vaccines. The HPV vaccine is the only one in U.S. history not to be approved for simultaneous distribution among male and female citizens alike. The approval of the HPV vaccine in 2006 reveals a particularly gendered moment in U.S. public health history because it presented the health condition, its complications, and its solution as a women's-only health issue. As such, public discourse surrounding HPV vaccination presents a particularly ripe opportunity to investigate gendered rhetorical practices central to constructing, managing, and constraining U.S. bodies at risk.

This chapter combines methods of discourse tracing (LeGreco and Tracy) and rhetorical analysis (Foss) to examine gendered policy, publicity, and practices surrounding the HPV vaccination. The goal is, first, to identify how HPV came to be defined as a woman-centered pathology in public health discourse, second, to describe for-profit mechanisms that designate women as the guardians of health not only for themselves and their families but also for the general U.S. public and, third, to explain how routine healthcare practices continue to normalize the gendering of this particular pathology in ways that ready female bodies for lifelong medical surveillance. Gendered approaches to medical intervention may limit the overall health of a population because they routinely and consistently affix the medical gaze upon the health of particular bodies rather than on the nature of disease. A relational framing of disease prevention may provide alternative strategies for public health policy, consumer public relations, and health care practices moving forward.

Public Health Rhetorics of HPV

According to the World Health Organization, HPV is the second-most-common cancer among women worldwide and is responsible for the death of 300,000 individuals annually (Rubin). Within the United States, HPV is the most common sexually transmitted infection (Satterwhite) and cervical cancer will strike about 11,500 women and claim an estimated 3,670 lives each year (Hendricks). Recognizing cervical cancer as an immediate and enduring threat, in 2006 U.S. public health officials moved quickly to approve and administer technology used to inhibit the spread of HPV, a virus causing 70% of all cases of cervical cancer (McClean). Transcripts from the vaccine's U.S. Food and Drug Administration (FDA) hearings, however, suggest that while the vaccine could have been approved for men and women, sexual and gendered ideologies regarding the female body led to its approval as an exclusively female vaccine (Thompson). Discourse surrounding HPV vaccination, therefore, presents a particularly gendered moment in health history and as such an opportunity to investigate the role of gender in American healthcare policy processes.

The gender component of Gardasil®, the brand name of the HPV vaccine, was criticized by early public commentators (Horton; Kessler and Wood), who pointed out that discussion about Gardasil® and HPV was shaped by assumptions about girls' and women's lives, rather than biological realities. In academic circles similar arguments have been made. Miriam Mara observes that "discussions about public health, which include multiple actors and narratives, at times focus the action toward female bodies" and that the HPV vaccine "[follows] these well-worn paths, which medicalize women's bodies and request or require medical treatments for women and girls that they might not otherwise choose" (125). Likewise, Marie Thompson argues that "issues of health related to cervical cancer are not solely situated with sexuality, but more often are further contextualized in frames of systematic regulation of women's bodies, in stigmatized, fossilized ideologies concerning women and sexuality" (128). Thompson warns that "the discursive manifestations of HPV and Gardasil® fail to fully include men or hold males to the standard of scrutiny their female counterparts endure" (127). This, in part, is caused by an overemphasis on the cervical consequence of HPV, the deemphasis of the sexual transmission of the virus, and the underreporting of the male role in the spread of the condition.

Likewise, a team of interdisciplinary scholars have more recently argued that gender norms across the realms of science, economics, and politics have systematically worked in concert to define HPV as a female-specific disease across time (Daley et al.). Examining the "interplay of science and sexism" (143) this team of medical professionals and social scientists conclude that HPV has indeed been "feminized," its social construction focused on females (142). Drawing from and adding to a line of critical and feminist scholarship with roots in poverty research specifically, the authors warn "feminization has the potential to negatively impact public awareness and approaches to address social and health issues across multiple stakeholder levels (e.g. governments, organizations)" (143). To better "face the issue of feminization of HPV directly," these authors advocate for a "multilevel approach in normalizing HPV vaccines as an important aspect of overall health for all individuals" (146).

In the following sections, I similarly trace HPV discourse across different realms to make sense of how and why HPV continues to be dubbed a women's-only health issue. Methodologically, "discourse tracing analyzes the formation, interpretation, and appropriation of discursive practices across micro, meso, and macro levels. In doing so, the method provides a language for studying social processes" (LeGreco and Tracy 1). Pairing archived historical events with rhetorical sensibilities allows me to draw attention to and interpret the specifically persuasive features of various discourses to explain how and why, in this particular case, certain social norms and expectations have come to accompany public perceptions of HPV, its causes, and its solution. Beyond advocating for the normalization of a gender-neutral vaccination, this type of rhetorically sensitive analysis reveals that a relational approach to HPV talk may further Daley et al.'s project and provide opportunities to address their concerns more readily. Specifically, addressing the relational dimensions of HPV transmission may help equip practitioners with models for thinking about and talking about vaccination beyond the particular patient (e.g. a method for sidestepping the "*my daughter isn't having sex*" standoff) and models for helping move our larger public health conversation beyond the male–female binary in ways that account for different types of coupling and care.

Direct-to-Consumer Advertisements and HPV

HPV gained widespread public recognition in March 2006 when the national "Tell Someone" campaign was launched by Merck, a pharmaceutical company exploring a cure, and the Cancer Society of America, raising awareness about cervical cancer (Whalen). The advertisements explicitly instructed viewers to "tell someone" about the link between a common virus (HPV) and cervical cancer. The U.S. Centers for Disease Control and Prevention (CDC) had long classified HPV as a sexually transmitted infection linked to cervical cancer in women, as well as head, neck, and anal cancer in men, and genital warts and less common forms of genital and oral cancers in both men and women (Dooren; Tuller). However, this early awareness campaign largely neglected the sexual nature of disease transmission and foregrounded the link between HPV and cervical cancer almost exclusively. Across the general U.S. public, since boys do not have cervixes, HPV thusly designated a women's-only health issue.

Later that same year, Merck's Gardasil® was approved by the U.S. Food and Drug Administration as the first vaccine to prevent infection by two strains of HPV responsible for 70% of all cases of cervical cancer, and two other strains responsible for about 90% of all cases of genital warts (CDC, "HPV Vaccine"). The quadrivalent HPV vaccine was only approved for use in "girls and women ages 9 through 26" (Rubin 8). Paired with early media coverage, the gender-specific FDA approval further convinced the general American public that HPV was/is a female-specific problem. Nearly six months after FDA approval of Gardasil®, in June 2006, Merck launched its second wave of advertising, "a national print, television and online advertising campaign for the world's first cervical cancer vaccine" ("Merck Launches"). This campaign continued to raise awareness about the link between this virus and cervical cancer (Whalen), relied heavily on emotional appeals associated with cancer, and never mentioned anything related to sexual transmission or the nature of the virus itself.

Dubbed "One Less," the second wave of Merck advertisements promoted Gardasil® as the method for eradicating cervical cancer. Building from the foundation laid by the previous "tell someone" awareness campaign this next wave of direct-to-consumer advertisements depicted mothers standing with daughters in matching T-shirts touting the campaign's slogan to ensure each vaccinated girl is "one less" cancer victim (Dederer). Notably, this campaign also emphasized the link between HPV and cervical cancer but excluded discussion of HPV as a sexually transmitted condition. In some ways defining HPV in terms of cervical cancer instead of in terms of sexual health anticipated pushback about protecting young girls (as early as 9 years of age) against a risk only introduced through sexual activity. In some extreme cases, parents worried that vaccinating girls might even encourage sexual behavior (see Malkowski, Renegar, and Dionisopoulos for details on this debate). Foregrounding the role of mothers across early advertisements may have intensified early concerns and backlash by affirming that HPV vaccinations were first and foremost a parenting decision, rather than a public health initiative.

Nonetheless, from the beginning, mothers were targeted as a central symbol of the fight against cervical cancer and this only continued through later iterations of the HPV vaccine and its campaigning. Motherhood and mothering serve as a prominent symbol used to help explain and control the threat of disease within the United States more widely and so, in many ways, it is unsurprising that this strategy appears across the rhetoric of HPV vaccination as well.

When boys became part of the Gardasil®'s target demographic in 2009, in many ways the formula for ushering them into the rhetoric of HPV vaccination was already in place. Instead of creating a new discourse about how HPV affects men and the transmission of the disease, the worst consequence of HPV (cancer) was once again emphasized and mothers were invoked as key decision makers for HPV vaccination. Although boys and fathers were now mentioned in HPV vaccine marketing efforts, the emphasis remained on girls, cervical cancer, and mothers.

Nearly a half a dozen years after the "One Less" campaign Merck launched another campaign that included boys and men as vaccine recipients. Unlike the first awareness campaign ("Tell Someone") and the Gardasil introduction campaign ("One Less") that were launched around the approval of the women-only Gardasil vaccine, this latest campaign came years after FDA approval of a version of the vaccine for men and boys. Immediately criticized for its overt emotional appeals directed at parents specifically (see McGinley), the advertisements told the story of two cancer victims in reverse chronological order. Beginning with the story of a young woman, the narrative unfolds through a series of photographs that start in the present with a woman stating "I have cervical cancer" and move back in time to conclude with a young girl asking "Did you know—Mom, Dad?". Immediately following that story, the commercial cuts to an orange screen with the following rhetorical question at center: "Who knew HPV could cause certain cancers and diseases in girls?" The next screen states: "And boys." And then, in the same reverse chronologically order, a visually driven narrative of a young man with cancer is told. Here too his adult voice over is used to explain facts about HPV before noting: "Maybe they didn't know I would end up with cancer because of HPV... Maybe if they had known there was a vaccine that could have protected me when I was 11 or 12. ... Maybe my parents just didn't know?" Followed by his on screen adolescent self asking: "Right Mom? Dad?"

The order of the stories depicted here—the woman's and then the man's—paired with the ordering of the parents mentioned—"mom" and then "dad"—subtly emphasize ongoing gendered understandings of the disease. Likewise, the omission of the exact type of cancer the young male character suffers juxtaposed against the very specific declarative statement offered by the female character ("I have cervical cancer") is noteworthy for the ways the ads once again sidestep addressing the male realities of HPV. Whereas significant strides were made in terms of depicting why men should care about HPV at an individual level, it still implicitly prioritized the female vaccine recipient (daughter), a certain type of advocate (mom), and a very specific type of cancer to be avoided (cervical). Additionally, as critics noted, the advertisement prioritized parents as its target audience and made exclusive use of emotional appeals centered on guilt and shame (Ramsey) rather than logical appeals focused on dispelling misconceptions about HPV and ushering boys and men into the conversation as equal participants that also needed to make up for lost time. Instead, the passivity of the male participant was reaffirmed in subtle ways, such as his use of the passive voice to speak about the threat of HPV that implicated others in his diagnosis and treatment ("maybe they didn't know I would end up with cancer"). This sharply contrasts with his female counterpart who spoke in an active, declarative manner ("I have cervical cancer") about the consequences of HPV.

HPV Healthcare Practices

When it comes to healthcare, in many ways American women are asked—and conditioned—to mitigate tensions between the "government's obligation to safeguard the health of its people and the rights of individuals to make their own decisions about matters affecting their health and their children" (Hendricks 1). Indeed, often within the American healthcare model, women are not only expected to act in their own best health-related interest, but they are also expected to be the custodians of health for men, children, and families (Miles; Sabo). Routine health care practices surrounding the Gardasil vaccination highlight how standard medical procedure instituted by this particular prevention technology shape relationships between women and medicine in socially consequential ways.

When the HPV vaccine was originally introduced, it required three office visits spread out over the course of six or more months wherein female vaccine recipients received one shot at each visit. The recommended vaccination age of 11–12 paired with this three-part vaccine schedule was intended to help maximize immunity for the individual vaccine recipient prior to HPV exposure through sexual activity: according to Eaton et al., 6.2% of adolescents nationwide initiate sexual activity prior to age 13. Although more recent versions of the vaccine require only two doses of the vaccine plus one recommended booster shot (CDC, "Clinician FAQ"), effectively completing the full vaccination series poses an ongoing challenge for public health officials. According to a 2016 national survey,

65% of girls aged 13–17 years had received at least one dose of the HPV vaccine but only 50% had received all doses in the series.

A multi-part vaccine sequence introduced at an age when adolescent girls are learning about what it means to be a responsible health participant routinizes medical interactions as a regular and necessary part of healthy citizenship. This is not to say that routine medical care is not valued as part of public life; it is to note that because girls were the only early vaccine recipients this three-part sequence implicitly communicated and behaviorally reinforced routine medical interactions as a regular and necessary part of healthy *female* citizenship. Additionally, the recommended timeline for introduction of the vaccine coincides with the average age U.S. women get their first period (Anderson, Dallal, and Must).

Women's sexual and reproductive health is embedded in patriarchal practices of medicine that exert subtle forms of control over women's bodies. Two modes of conditioning that situate women as key campaigners of public health arise from the female menstrual cycle specifically (the epitome of woman, see Peake, Manderson, and Potts). First, upon getting their period and/or becoming sexually active women are taught that annual Pap smear exams, and thus routinized interactions with healthcare, are expected. Second, women are taught that motherhood and the ability to bear children signify womanhood. As a result of the equation of womanhood with motherhood, women become part of a system of regular health examinations. The alignment of the HPV vaccination schedule with physical signifiers of womanhood may only work to solidify these assumptions. In and of itself, this may not necessarily be problematic, but what is troubling is that few routine practices exist for adolescent boys to equivalently prepare men for routine medical interactions as central to public health participation.

For example, the *Journal of the American Medical Association* has reported that women ages 20 to 24 have the highest overall prevalence of HPV, and that prevalence increases each year from ages 14 to 24 (Tuller). By contrast, the prevalence of HPV in men cannot be fully ascertained because, to-date, no HPV test exists for men (CDC, "Genital HPV"): "The only approved HPV tests on the market are for screening women for cervical cancer. They are not useful for screening for HPV-related cancers or genital warts in men" (CDC, "Vaccine Information"). A man usually finds out he has HPV when he has an outbreak. Many strains of HPV, including the cervical-cancer-causing strains, do not cause visible outbreaks. Women may have the highest overall prevalence of HPV, but then again they are the only ones being proactively tested. Consent with medical processes is often gained through the invocation of symbolic devices used to resonate with already established common-sense ideologies embedded in discourse (Gamson and Modigliani). For the case of HPV, testing further symbolizes routine medical surveillance as a practice of healthy female citizenship.

Working in concert with larger American ideologies that tout individual choice, Public Health runs the risk of creating a situation where individual women who cannot get vaccinated or tested, who choose not to get vaccinated and contract cervical cancer years from now, or who get tested and are unable to adequately do anything with that information, may be blamed for their condition: "Such concerns about victim-blaming are particularly pertinent in this area, given that there are no straightforward behavioural choices that can be recommended to guarantee absolute protection from the sexual transmission of HPV" (Braun and Gavey 1472). It becomes the role of health scholars and advocates alike, then, to expose gendered practices in medicine in order to evaluate their use on the larger scale of public health. Adding men to the rhetoric of HPV as partners and stakeholders will not only work to alleviate the burden of public health that has fallen on women, but it will also work to expedite our joint goal of a world free of (cervical) cancer.

Implications

HPV, like other communicable diseases, does not recognize gender as an organizing principle but instead reminds us of the intersections between medicine, health, and a larger American public. Furthermore, HPV reminds us of the various ways we are connected to one another in social and biological senses. The vaccination discourse detailed in this analysis highlights the persuasive capacities of pharmaceutical rhetoric and health care practices to emphasize the social and political responsibilities assumed with shaping discourses and practices of health and medicine at a public level. With regard to the larger field of Public Health, these findings enhance our understanding of the ways that rhetoric contributes to the trajectory of medical interventions and, likely, the overall success of disease prevention efforts on a national scale.

In order for vaccinations to be successful, they require that the large majority of a population become vaccinated. "Herd immunity," a phenomenon that requires a certain percentage (ideally 80%) of a given population be vaccinated in order to protect the unvaccinated among them (Fine, Eames, and Heymann), is an essential component of disease eradication. Partial vaccination undermines the opportunity for a population to adequately manage a disease because it may work to counteract initiatives underway and cause a particular vaccine to be deemed a failure even when the science on that vaccine is sound.

In order for the HPV vaccine to succeed, both men and women need to experience a significant rise in disease resistance or the overall population will continue to face complications and consequences caused by the condition. In order to achieve this goal, new strategies for talking about the spread of HPV, the consequences related to HPV, and the responsibility and accountability associated with eliminating HPV are required. Focusing on the relational dimension of disease transmission may present one strategy for doing so, an approach that has been notably absent from HPV messaging thus far.

Relational Approaches to Public Health Messaging

Early definitions of the health threat and promotion of a gender-specific cure skewed vaccination trends in ways that continue to impact how/if boys and men enter the conversation. From the beginning, a gender-neutral HPV vaccine would have been desirable for a few reasons: HPV can cause genital warts, and head, neck, and anal cancer in men; and, preventing infection in boys could also help reduce the rate of infection in women because men transmit HPV to women (Dooren; Tuller). During the first few years of the national HPV awareness campaign boys and men were officially excluded from the HPV discussion thus gendering HPV's image as a feminine disease. Since then, boys and men have been secondarily addressed at best. Not only do more concerted efforts need to be made to foreground men's roles in HPV prevention, alternative models for talking about HPV need to emerge to help blur the binary between men and women altogether. It seems that, unlike other vaccinations, the rhetorical history of HPV has been indelibly marred by a men-versus-women framing. In order to undo this past, perhaps, an altogether alternative approach to public health messaging is warranted.

Relationships hold significant sense-making value among both men and women and so a relational approach to public health messaging about this particular condition could encourage shared responsibility for HPV prevention and management. Positivistic science may not prioritize how relationships factor into medicine. However, as more and more literature pressures key policy makers and health advocates to consider relational dynamics of epidemiology, the field of health is experiencing sustained curiosity with regard to modes of feasible prevention. HPV vaccination operates as a case study for the ways that gender and biology go head-to-head in a battle to define public health. The solution will require both a social and a biological component. Sex does indeed serve a biological function; however, sex also serves social and relational dimensions of health. The relational aspect of disease transmission may present a new opportunity for thinking through and shaping HPV talk and HPV prevention.

As bioethicist Donna Dickenson's book title—*Me Medicine vs. We Medicine: Reclaiming Biotechnology for the Common Good* (2016)—communicates we have entered an era of "Me Medicine" at the expense of "We Medicine," a trend with significant consequences especially with regard to vaccination technologies. Conceptualizing public health, however, requires individuals to understand how they are connected to others. Ongoing disregard for the relational dynamics of health fails to tap into a sense-making structure already in place that could be used to transfer knowledge and influence across the U.S. population at the intimate, dyadic level. The impersonal depiction of HPV transmission specifically has allowed audiences to more readily focus on the biology of cervical cancer as opposed to the precursory virus and, thus, further a sex binary when it comes to the management of this disease in particular. Since the HPV vaccine has now been approved for both females and males it means that across various types of couples and coupling HPV prevention can and should become a topic of conversation. Public health promotion campaigns influence how these types of conversations can occur by modeling and promoting ideal health behaviors. When it comes to disease management, communicating with others openly and earnestly about prevention options *is* an ideal public health practice, one that requires individuals to understand how their own health status intersects with the statuses of others. In terms of its public image and its implementation of practice, HPV rhetoric ignores the fact that protection from sexually-transmitted diseases and cervical cancer requires more than just a vaccine, it requires interpersonal communication about risks that affect us all.

Conclusions

When Gardasil gained FDA approval, the deputy secretary of the Department of Health and Human Services at that time released a statement claiming that Gardasil was "a major step forward in public health protection," (Rubin 4) and that due to the vaccine "we can now include the worst types of HPV and most cervical cancer among the diseases that no one need suffer and die from" (Gellene A4). However, more than a decade after its FDA approval and introduction to the market a world free of cervical cancer may still be a long time coming. This chapter offers a vision for what is at stake, from an institutional perspective, in perpetuating gendered communication to promote public health. Although the condition of cervical cancer is in itself inextricably gendered, modes of HPV prevention need not be.

In December 2014 the FDA approved GARDASIL 9®, a second-generation vaccine that prevents nine types of HPV including seven strains linked to cancers. This vaccine was approved for use in females 9–26 years of age and for males ages 9–15 years. Almost exactly one year later, the FDA expanded that age bracket to include 16–26-year-old males as well and in October 2016 the CDC officially added the HPV vaccine to the list of recommended "routine vaccinations" for both girls and boys ages 11–12 years old. Despite these gender-neutralizing moves, HPV vaccine uptake remains lower among boys and men than girls and women. Specifically, a national survey conducted in 2016 found that 50% of girls aged 13–17 years had completed their HPV vaccine series as compared to only 38% of boys in that same age bracket (Walker et al.). Discrepancies in vaccination uptake can be attributed, at least in part, to the residual effects of early, gendered HPV rhetoric. Alternative HPV messaging that pivots on the social dimensions of disease transmission rather than the biological realities of disease outcomes could expand the audience for HPV vaccinations and, perhaps more importantly, could redistribute the burden of disease across the U.S. population writ large, rather than focusing on women specifically.

Works Cited

AndersonSarah E., Gerard E. Dallal, and Aviva Must. "Relative Weight and Race Influence Average Age at Menarche: Results from Two Nationally Representative Surveys of US Girls Studied 25 Years Apart." *Pediatrics* 111. 4 Pt 1 (April 2003): 844–850.

Bordo, Susan. *Unbearable Weight: Feminism, Western Culture and the Body.* Berkeley: University of California Press, 2004

Braun, Virginia and Nicola Gavey. "'With the Best of Reasons': Cervical Cancer Prevention Policy and the Suppression of Sexual Risk Factor Information." *Social Science and Medicine* 48(1999): 1463–1474.

CDC (Centers for Disease Control and Prevention). "Clinician FAQ: CDC Recommendations for HPV Vaccine 2-Dose Schedules." National Center for Immunization and Respiratory Diseases. 30 November 2016. www.cdc.gov/hpv/downloads/HCVG15-PTT-HPV-2Dose.pdf.

CDC. "Genital HPV Infection – CDC Fact Sheet." National Center for HIV/AIDS, Viral Hepatitis, STD, and TB Prevention. July2017. www.cdc.gov/std/hpv/hpv-Fs-July-2017.pdf.

CDC. "HPV Vaccine Questions and Answers." August 2006. www.cdc.gov/std/hpv/STDFact-HPV-vaccine.html.

CDC. "Vaccine Information Statement: HPV Vaccine; What You Need to Know" (Report 42 U.S.C. 300aa-26). 2012. www.cdc.gov/vaccines/hcp/vis/current-vis.html.

Daley, Ellen M., Cheryl A. Vamos, Erika L. Thompson, Gregory D. Zimet, Zeev Rosberger, Laura Merrell, and Nolan S. Kline. "The Feminization of HPV: How Science, Politics, Economics and Gender Norms Shaped U.S. HPV Vaccine Implementation." *Papillomavirus Research* 3(2017): 142–148.

Dederer, Claire. "Pitching Protection to Both Mothers and Daughters." *New York Times*18 February2007. www.nytimes.com/2007/02/18/arts/television/18dede.html.

Dickinson, Donna. *Me Medicine vs. We Medicine: Reclaiming Biotechnology for the Common Good.* New York: Columbia University Press, 2016.

Dooren, J. C. "Merck Cervical-Cancer Vaccine is Approved for Use in Women: Gardasil Could Sharply Cut Key Viruses Behind Disease; CDC to Set Forth Guidelines." *Wall Street Journal* 9 June 2006: A16.

Eaton, Danice K., Laura Kann, Steve Kinchen, Shari Shanklin, Katherine H. Flint, Joseph Hawkins, et al. "Youth Risk Behavior Surveillance—United States, 2011." *Morbidity and Mortality Weekly Report Surveillance Summaries* 61. 4(2012): 1–162.

Fine, Paul, Ken Eames, and David L. Heymann. "'Herd Immunity': A Rough Guide." *Clinical Infectious Diseases* 52(2011): 911–916.

Foss, Sonia K. *Rhetorical Criticism: Exploration and Practice.* Long Grove: Waveland, 2004.

Gamson, William A. "A Constructionist Approach to Mass Media and Public Opinion." *Symbolic Interaction* 11(1988): 161–174.

Gamson, W.A. and A. Modigliani. "Media Discourse and Public Opinion: A Constructionist Approach." *American Journal of Sociology* 95(1989): 1–37.

Gellene, Denise. "Panel Wants Vaccine to be Routine: All 11- and 12-year-old Girls Would Get Shots Against Cervical Cancer. Some Conservatives Oppose a Mandate: States Will Have to Decide." *Los Angeles Times* 30 June 2006: A18.

Hendricks, Melissa. "HPV Vaccine: Who Chooses?: Because Immunization Can Prevent Cervical Cancer, Bills Seek to Mandate Shots. Some Say Such Measures are Ethically Suspect." *Los Angeles Times* 5 February 2007: F1.

Horton, Mary Jane. "A Shot Against Cervical Cancer: A Stunning New Youth Vaccine Promises to Prevent the Deadly Disease—But Will Parents Go for It?" *Ms. Magazine.* www.msmagazine.com/summer2005/cervicalcancer.asp.

Kessler, Bree and Summer Wood. "A Shot in the Dark: What—and Who—is Behind the Marketing of GARDASIL®?" *Ms. Magazine* 36(2007): 27–28, 32.

LeGreco, Marianne and Sarah J. Tracy. "Discourse Tracing as Qualitative Practice." *Qualitative Inquiry* 15(2009): 1516–1543.

Lorber, Judith. "Believing is Seeing: Biology as Ideology." *Gender and Society* 7(1993): 568–581.

Malkowski, J.A., V.R. Renegar, and G.N. Dionisopoulos. "The HPV Mandatory Vaccination Controversy: Creating a Frame of Perspective for Public Health Initiatives." *Contemporary Case Studies in Health Communication: Theoretical and Applied Approaches*. Ed. M. Brann. Thousand Oaks, CA: Sage, 2015. 337–350.

Mara, Miriam. "Spreading the (Dis)ease: Gardasil and the Gendering of HPV." *Feminist Formations* 22(2011): 124–143.

McClean, V. "Rush to Require Cancer Shot Threatens to Promote Backlash." *USA Today* 9 February 2007: A14.

McGinley, Laurie. "Do the New Merck HPV Ads Guilt-trip Parents or Tell Hard Truths? Both." *The Washington Post* 11 August 2016.

Medical News Today. "Merck Launches National Advertising Campaign for Gardasil, Merck's New Cervical Cancer Vaccine." *Medical News Today* 23 November 2006. www.medicalnewstoday.com.

Miles, Agnes. *Women, Health and Medicine*. Buckingham: Open UP, 1991.

Peake, Susan, Lenore Manderson, and Helen Potts. "'Part and Parcel of Being a Woman': Female Urinary Incontinence and Constructions of Control." *Medical Anthropology Quarterly* 13(1999): 267–285.

Ramsey, Lydia. "A Shocking New Ad is Shaming Parents for Not Giving their Children this Unpopular Vaccine." *Business Insider* 15 July 2016.

Rubin, Rita. "First-Ever Cancer Vaccine Approved." *USA Today* 8 June 2006. www.usa today.com.

Sabo, Don. "Men's Health Studies: Origins and Trends." *Journal of American College Health* 49(2000): 133–142.

Satterwhite, Catherine L., Elizabeth Torrone, Elissa Meites, et al. "Sexually Transmitted Infections Among US Women and Men: Prevalence and Incidence Estimates, 2008." *Sexually Transmitted Diseases* 40. 3(2013): 187–193.

Thompson, Marie. "Who's Guarding What? A Poststructural Feminist Analysis of Gardasil Discourses." *Health Communication* 25. 2(2010): 119–130.

Tuller, David. "New Vaccine for Cervical Cancer Could Prove Useful in Men, Too." *New York Times* 30 January 2007. www.nytimes.com/2007/01/30/health/30virus.html.

Walker, Tanja Y., Laurie D. Elam-Evans, James A. Singleton, et al. "National, Regional, State, and Selected Local Area Vaccination Coverage Among Adolescents Aged 13–17 Years—United States, 2016." *Morbidity and Mortality Weekly Report* 66. 33(2017): 874–882.

West, Candace and Don H. Zimmerman. "Doing Gender." *Gender and Society* 1. 2(June 1987): 125–151.

Whalen, Jeanne. "Armed with New Vaccines, Drug Makers Target Teenagers." *Wall Street Journal* 23 August 2006: B1.

Wharton, Amy S. *The Sociology of Gender: An Introduction to Theory and Research*. Chichester: Wiley-Blackwell, 2012.

9 Bacteriology and Modernity
Phenomenology, Biopolitics, Ontology

Jens Lohfert Jørgensen

Around 1900, bacteriology offered a new interpretation of the relationship between the individual and the surrounding world, problematizing existing notions about humanity and contributing to the formation of new ones. Growing public awareness about the ability of para- or under-phenomenal organisms to colonize the body and to proliferate within it prepared the ground for a bacillophobia, exacerbated by hygiene campaigns. By demonstrating that we exist in close symbiosis with a seething multitude of non-human organisms, however, this awareness also challenged the anthropocentric world view that had dominated since the Enlightenment. As a symbolic form, the interaction between the human body and bacteria articulated the relation between interior and exterior on a perspectival scale ranging from the individual to the global. Thus, bacteria were used conceptually to make sense of a rapidly-changing world, as reflected in the literature of the day. I posit that the "bacterial focus" on a changing world moved the work of prominent authors towards what can be termed an embodied modernism. From a phenomenological, biopolitical, and ontological perspective, I focus on three literary works written at the turn of the twentieth century and their depiction of the interplay between bacillophobia and a dawning post-anthropocentrism.

Bacillophobia

As medical historian David S. Barnes notes, germ theory at once changed medicine fundamentally, and, on another level, not at all (2). In the 1870s, medical practitioners and observers believed that diseases were caused by heredity, climate, miasmas, and immoderate lifestyles. Although experts agreed that the presence of living microorganisms was the essential condition for infection by the mid-1890s,[1] therapeutic measures against diseases changed very little. Treatments continued to correspond to older etiological views, targeting the manifest symptoms of disease, and were primarily palliative.

Compared to earlier theories, bacteriology had a specifying effect on the etiology and the diagnosis of diseases: in contrast to more abstract phenomena, bacteria were quantifiable, and their appearance, features, and life-span were determinable (Vigarello 203). But this knowledge depended on advanced technology. For the public, bacteriology challenged the commonsensical notion that the causes of disease are directly perceptible via one or more senses. To the naked eye, bacteria are paraphenomenal: insensuous phenomena that exist in the realm of the sensuous. They are, so to speak, under-phenomenal. Amongst the public, this gap between theoretical knowledge and common sense experience created a marked anxiety about the threat posed by bacteria. Hygiene campaigns only exacerbated this anxiety. Whereas prior pathogenic factors were seen as passive and inert, bacteria were depicted as more powerful, more aggressive, and more destructive than any hitherto known disease-provoking agent.

A general social-hygienic tendency around the turn of the century was to anthropomorphize bacteria, attributing a malign intentionality to them. The ability of invisible germs to invade the body was emphasized, "ever ready to step in and take possession of the body" (Cromie 133). Invasion was highly likely, since bacteria are omnipresent: "the hostile microbe is in fact every-where—within and without us, seeking, we might say, what it might devour" (Capitan 107). The damage caused by bacteria was also irreversible, due to their incredible pathogenicity: "If an opening appears on the outside, these microbes penetrate the structure and it takes only a few hours, in some cases, to destroy even the strongest system" (Dujardin-Beaumetz, quoted in Vigarello 205). Finally, the fecundity of germs was emphasized:

> They multiply with such rapidity ... that, according to the calculations of an eminent biologist, a single one must, if the proper conditions could be maintained, in less than five days generate a mass that would fill the space occupied by all the oceans on the earth's surface, supposing these to have an average depth of one mile.
>
> (Parke 168)

Statements like this served as optimum facilitators of bacteriological anxiety in the public consciousness. In the 1906 Swedish novel *Doctor Glas*, Hjalmar Söderberg describes a man suffering from "the disease referred to as bacillopho-bia" (86), that is, a meta-disease. Bacteriology certainly participated in the "dis-enchantment" of the world that Max Weber saw as characteristic of modernity (13–14). But expressions of bacillophobia demonstrate an ambiguous tendency and testify to a re-enchanted fear that nature might not be controllable after all.[2]

Phenomenology

Bacteriology thus contributed to the altered phenomenology of modernity. In 1884, physicist and philosopher Ernst Mach formulated a radical version of this phe-nomenology, describing the physical world as consisting of unstable compounds of sense data: "Colors, sounds, temperatures, pressures, spaces, time and so forth, are connected with one another in manifold ways; and with them are associated dis-positions of mind, feelings, and volitions" (2). In this view, phenomena are made up solely of these sense data, which are in a state of constant flux, offering no fixed points of orientation. Similarly, man lacks a stable self, and changes according to the shifting sensory impressions issued from his surroundings.

In a related vein, Henri Lefebvre describes how, around 1900, the "referentials broke down one after another under the influence of various pressures (science, technology and social changes)" (112). Electricity and unprecedented speed, for instance, changed the perception of outlines and motion respectively, and the relationships between oppositional, independent absolutes such as light/ darkness and stasis/mobility became relative. The sensory apparatus thus underwent a development from immediacy to abstraction. As Lefebvre puts it, the senses became "theoreticians" (113). This development heralded a rupture between conventional and specialized sensation, and sensory principles previously considered permanent and universal began to disintegrate. By virtue of the challenge they posed to the senses, bacteria disclosed this rupture.

One possible approach to literary works that deal with the altered phenomenology of modernity is so-called cultural phenomenology as formulated by scholars such as Steven Connor and David Trotter. As the designation implies, cultural phenomenology attempts to establish a dialogue between the understanding of artifacts and practices in cultural studies as mediations of discourses, on the one hand, and, on the other, the attempt of phenomenology to articulate the embodied character of the subject's experience of the world. I refer primarily to the phenomenological thinking of Maurice Merleau-Ponty here. According to him, what underlies our objective, intellectual experience of the world is a mute corporeal knowledge of so-called pre-objective phenomena. The body opens itself to these emerging and ambiguous phenomena via the sensorium. It is "the vehicle for being in the world" (94).

Joris-Karl Huysmans' novel *À rebours* (1884), translated variously as *Against the Grain* or *Against Nature*, [3] can be read as a staging of the contribution of bacteriology to the altered phenomenology of modernity. The novel is often characterized as a "paradigm," a "manifesto," or an "encyclopedia" of *fin-de-siècle* cultural decadence (Weir 83, 97). It depicts the refined and hypersensitive Duc Jean Des Esseintes' endeavour to isolate himself completely in a house in Fontenay outside Paris, in reaction to what he experiences as the unrest, filthiness, and vulgarity of modern society. His figure thus incarnates an adherence to Friedrich Nietzsche's notion of solitude as hygienic, since "all contact between man and man—in 'society'—must inevitably be unclean" (195). Such isolation can be related to Georges Vigarello's observation that, for the first time in history, the break-through of the germ theory of disease caused hygienic ideals to point "to a perfection perpetually beyond reach" (204).

This relation between solitude and hygiene is developed in *À rebours* through Des Esseintes' isolation, as he attempts to regain the sensory self-control that he has, in society, experienced the loss of. The novel consists mainly of hyperdetailed descriptions of how he carefully furnishes his house with a view to creating quite specific sensational and emotional effects, thereby creating an artificial sensory universe of which he is the sovereign. The attempt, however, is in vain. Traversing these descriptive passages, the narrative depicts the gradual disintegration of Des Esseintes' self control, thereby of his hygienic-solitary ideal. This process is caused by an accretion of factors. First, the state of isolation itself proves increasingly problematic as it aggravates rather than improves Des Esseintes' exhaustion. Second, he faces external impulses in the form of the acute effects on the senses to which he exposes himself. Third, internal impulses build up during his isolation. Here, I will discuss an example of these internal impulses in the awakening of Des Esseintes' latent religious faith.

Des Esseintes' attraction to religion, *in casu* Catholicism, dates from his school days in a Jesuit monastery. There, the teachers succeeded in "implanting particular ideas" in the students (Huysmans, Against Nature 63). Huysmans' original novel employs pictorial language that merges botanical and bacterial metaphors to account for the development of Des Esseintes' faith. This ambiguity is obscured in Margaret Mauldon's otherwise excellent English translation: "implanting," translated from "greffer" (Huysmans, À rebours 77), elides the French meaning "to inoculate" which also means "to impregnate (a person or animal) with the virus or germs of a disease." Huysmans describes how Des Esseintes had earlier been "resistant" (63) to these ideas, but now, due to his reading of Catholic works and the general monastic atmosphere of his existence, this resistance "was beginning to be eroded" (66) and a religious longing, which he had carried within him as an "unfermented leaven" (65), "slowly and obscurely ramified in his soul" (66). The reference to fermentation processes evokes Louis Pasteur's initial work on bacteria, which demonstrated that yeast comprises living microorganisms and not chemical compounds.

The bacteriological metaphors become more pronounced in the passage until the signs of Catholicism are simply referred to as "morbid symptoms" (67). In this constellation of references, the depiction of the awakening of Des Esseintes' faith corresponds quite accurately to the nature of endospores, the dormant, highly viable form to which certain bacteria can reduce themselves under environmental stress. In favorable conditions, the endospore is retransformed into a vegetative bacterium in three stages, namely activation, germination, and, finally, outgrowth (Bauman 545–552, 783–784).

Thus, what was originally conceived as a hermetically sealed, sterile exile proves to be the incubator for cultures of disease, both metaphorically and literally. Des Esseintes becomes increasingly physically and mentally exhausted. At the novel's conclusion, a doctor orders him to leave the house in Fontenay and return to Paris, where, ironically, he has to submit to "new hygienic conditions."[4] In the doctor's reaction, Huysmans elegantly illustrates a societal perspective where the primary concern is less the threat to his own well-being posed by Des Esseintes' neurosis than the socially subversive potential of his deviant life-style. The doctor emphasizes that Des Esseintes must resign himself to "ordinary life," and must "try to enjoy himself ... like other people" (173).

Biopolitics

Bacteria had a major conceptual impact on culture, functioning as what Ernst Cassirer calls "a symbolic form", that is, as a historically and culturally determined mental model that creates an image of reality by enabling a grasp of diverse sensory data as manageable totalities (Cassirer; Tygstrup and Holm 153–157). As a symbolic form, bacteria were drawn upon to describe the relationship between interiority and exteriority on the individual, societal, and even global levels. They were used in the attempt to comprehend a changing world, not only phenomenologically, but also socially and politically.

The figurative use of bacteria had biopolitical implications. This is perhaps unremarkable in light, on the one hand, of the alliance between bacteriology and established hygiene movements (Latour) and, on the other, the hygienic connotations of the concept of biopolitics, as it emerges in Michel Foucault's analyses of the governance of sexuality in eighteenth-century Europe (Prozorov and Rentea 1). Since *The Will to Knowledge* (1976), Foucault's notion of biopolitics has been further developed by several thinkers, amongst them Roberto Esposito. He relates biopolitics to the bacteria-relevant concepts of community and immunity. Drawing on Latin origins, Esposito notes that community membership means renouncing individual identity, as a duty and a gift, in "a progressive process to openness to the other-than-self" (84). Immunity, conversely, refers to a situation that cancels this renunciation, as is evident when the term is used in the juridical, as well as in the medical context. When individuals possess immunity or become immune, they are cut off from their surroundings. Mechanisms of immunity are necessary to preserve life, but Esposito points out that beyond a certain threshold, immunity not only protects the individual or social body but also prevents its development: "immunization at high doses is the sacrifice of the living—of every qualified life, that is—for the sake of mere survival. It is the reduction of life to bare biological matter" (85).

The concept of biopolitics is distended between two incompatible poles: on the one hand, a restraining and sometimes even apocalyptic form, and, on the other, a liberating and sometimes even euphoric form. According to Esposito, the restraining interpretation refers not to the subjugation of an external power over life, but to life's endeavour to defend itself against dangers via an immunization that contradicts other needs. What characterizes the intensification of biopolitics in modernity is a pull towards such an immunization of life that makes it an object of politics. In order to turn life into the subject of politics, Esposito encourages us "to overturn in some way—indeed in every way—the balance of power between 'common' and 'immune'; to separate the immunitary protection of life from its destruction by means of the common" (87–88). The common differs, on the one hand, from the private, and on the other, from the public. What is common is everybody's and nobody's: it does not belong to individual owners, and it does not belong to the state. It is a juridically undecided zone between the private and the public that has been diminished in modernity.

Esposito's notion of biopolitics is relevant to Joseph Conrad's 1897 novel *The Nigger of the "Narcissus"*, which depicts the voyage of a merchant vessel from Bombay to London. The ship's crew comprises twenty-six men, including eighteen so-called "foremast hands." One of them is a big, West Indian sailor,

James Wait. From the moment he is introduced, the narrator points the reader's attention to the way in which his performance of health affects the environment:

> He put his hand to his side and coughed twice, a cough metallic, hollow, and tremendously loud; it resounded like two explosions in a vault; the dome of the sky rang to it, and the iron plates of the ship's bulwarks seemed to vibrate in unison.
>
> (Conrad 11)

Wait performs his duties reluctantly and badly. After a week, he states that his lack of energy is caused by the wasting of his lungs (that is, by tuberculosis), and he is sent off to the forecastle. The enclosed space of the *Narcissus* is characterized by a static, increasingly charged atmosphere, whose main source is the long-standing insecurity regarding Wait's health. Is he a dying man or is he a "black fraud" (25), as his shipmate Donkin claims?[5]

Irrespective of whether the crew perceives of his weakness as real or pretended, Wait dominates the *Narcissus* with it and profits by it unscrupulously. His presence on the ship thus assumes a parasitical form, mirroring the presence of *mycobacterium tuberculosis* in his body. Wait challenges clear divisions between strength and disability, between independence and reliance, and, ultimately, between reality and appearance. Above all, he figures as a principle of ambivalence in *The Nigger of the "Narcissus"*. As the ship makes its way from India to England, the crew is infected by this ambivalence: "a black mist emanated from him; a subtle and dismal influence; a something cold and gloomy that floated out and settled on all the faces like a mourning veil" (21). His influence on the surroundings assumes an almost physical form that taints the atmosphere on board.

Life on the *Narcissus* is characterized by a detailed regimentation which has the production of value as its goal. The crew is, so to speak, owned by the ship during the journey. Following Esposito's line of thinking, the biopolitical cohesive force of the ship is the attempt to immunize the *Narcissus* against the dangers that threaten it, primarily in the shape of natural forces. This immunizing endeavor is necessary, of course, but as Esposito remarks, it also reduces life to bare biological matter. In taking on a restraining form, it corresponds to the negative interpretation of biopolitics. In opposition to this endeavor, Wait's ambivalent performance of his health can be understood as biopolitical in the positive sense, in that it takes on a liberating form. His infection of the crew takes the shape of a humanization that clashes with the hard discipline aboard the ship: "He was immortalising. Through him we were becoming highly humanised, tender, complex, excessively decadent" (85). The humanity with which he infects the crew causes them to risk their own well-being and the well-being of the ship for his. At any hour of the day or night, they assemble in his cabin, where he, and not the *Narcissus*, is the new focus of their attentive gaze. Thus, Wait functions as what Esposito calls a common good: due to his ambivalence, he evades the singular ownership of the ship; and this evasion makes him the subject of the crew's common ownership. He is everybody's and nobody's, a site of openness to "the other-than-self." In this sense, he turns the crew of the *Narcissus* into a community that is bound together by his infection of it.

Ontology

In its depiction of the relationship between John Wait and the crew on the *Narcissus*, Conrad's novel presents its readers with a conception of humanity that transgresses individualism and distances itself from anthropocentrism. Not only does the bacteria/body relationship serve as a symbolic form; it also has ontological implications for the conceptualization of the nature of humanity as such. These implications have recently been addressed by both philosophers and social scientists. The Canadian environmental scholar Myra J. Hird's concept of "microontologies" is a strong plea for a view of bacteria that moves beyond passive and pathogenic characterizations. The concept refers to an "ethics that engages seriously with the microcosmos" (Hird 1) of bacterial life in order to reconsider our approach to social topics. Her book *The Origins of Sociable Life* explores the challenge posed by contemporary scientific debates about bacteria to prevailing understandings of subjects such as evolution, identity, sex, and ecology.

One of these debates concerns endosymbiont theory, which has gained ground within biology over the last forty years. Endosymbionts are unicellular organisms that live in the cells of other organisms and benefit both. Thus, eukaryotes—organisms whose cells have a true nucleus—developed via a symbiotic relationship to prokaryotes—organisms whose cells lack a nucleus, such as bacteria. This hypothesis may suggest that the main principle behind the evolution of life is not the survival of the fittest organism but interaction and mutual dependence between organisms with entirely unrelated genomes. According to the prominent proponents of this theory, Lynn Margulis and Dorion Sagan, "[l]ife did not take over the globe by combat, but by networking" (29).

Hird discusses biological models of the self developed by evolutionary theory, including the "immunological individualism" implicit in virologist Frank Burnet's definition of immunity. This definition is based on a sharp differentiation between exogenous (or external) elements that trigger an immune reaction, and endogenous (or internal) elements that do not (usually); that is, a differentiation between non-self and self. Drawing on endosymbiont theory, Hird offers an alternative understanding. In a human body, 10% of cells are eukaryotic and 90% are bacteria; therefore, "any given human body is ... a symbiont" (84). As philosopher and science historian Alfred I. Tauber points out, this has serious implications for "immunological individualism." Exogenous elements do not necessarily trigger an immune reaction in an organism. On the contrary, the immune system "ignores much of what it sees. It allows the organism to engage its environment ...: the self/nonself border is ever-changing" (quoted in Hird 85). Hird concludes that "we are not autonomous individuals who subsequently interact ... we intra-act ..., and this ongoing process *creates* something we call individuality, to be re-created with every encounter" (88–89; italics in the original).

Hird's interest in the ontological implications of the bacteria/body relationship is anticipated by Mark Twain in his unfinished novel *3,000 Years Among the Microbes* (1905). The rather curious premise of the novel's plot is that its first-person narrator Huck is transformed into a cholera bacterium as a consequence of a magician's failed experiment and is subsequently introduced into the body of a vagabond. Here, Huck establishes an institute, which specializes in teaching ethics. As indicated by its title, the novel is presented as an investigation of bacterial life from Huck's personal perspective, translated "from the Original Microbic" by Mark Twain (433). The social organization of the bacteria in the vagabond's body has parallels to the organization of human beings: they speak different languages, have different nationalities and belong to different social classes. A similar parallelism applies to their self-conception: "The microbe's name for himself is ... *sooflasky*," which means "what the word Man—as chief creature in the scheme of Creation—means in the human World" (439; italics in the original).

3,000 Years Among the Microbes satirizes topical subjects in the U.S.A. of its day, such as the Christian Science movement and the annexation of the Philippines. But it also raises more universal questions regarding social conditions, morality, and anthropocentrism. This thematic diversity is balanced by one pervasive narrative technique, the doubling of the narrator's point of view. Although Huck quickly becomes bacteriologically naturalized, he also preserves his human consciousness. Twain uses the elasticity of his main character's perspective to address the habitus of humanity *in toto*. For example, species separatism, scaled down to a bacterial perspective, is taken up in relation to a theological discussion: are animals resurrected on the Day of Judgment, and if so, which ones?[6] Is it even the case for the "swinks," nanoscopic organisms that inhabit the bodies of the sooflaskies? An outside expert—a trypanosomiasis bacterium well studied in bacteriology as well as theology—makes it clear that nanoscopic organisms are indeed included. If any species deserves redemption, it is the swinks, due to their relentless but overlooked efforts to uphold the life of sooflaskies.

As a consequence of this conclusion, Huck experiences an epiphanic insight into the nature of the relationship between species, an insight that depends on the doubling of his perspective:

> The inexorable logic of the situation is this: there being a Man, with a Microbe to infest him, and for him to be indifferent about; and there being a Sooflasky, with a Swink to infest him, and for him to be indifferent about: then it follows, for a certainty, that the swink is similarly infested, too, and has something to look down upon and be indifferent to and sponge out upon occasion ...—and so on down and down till you strike the bottommost bottom of created life—if there is one, which is extremely doubtful.
>
> (527)

3,000 Years Among the Microbes can be read as a conceptual work, and its core concept is this *matryoshkan* vision of life that opens both upwards and downwards in dizzying scale *ad infinitum*. Twain formulated the idea in a notebook entry twenty years before he sat down to work on the novel. The vision's alienating exhibition of species separatism invites transgression of the very same separatism, exactly because it is depicted as a general condition. The notion that they are different to all other species is paradoxically what unites the species, and Huck's awareness of this relativizes the notion. This relativization is shared by current thinking on the implications of the bacteria/body relationship. All life forms are folded into each other in *3,000 Years Among the Microbes*; in Hird's terms, they intra-act.

Conclusion

Drawing on Robert Mitchell's differentiation between various conceptions of experimentation in the contexts of the histories of science and aesthetics, *Against Nature*, *The Nigger of the "Narcissus"*, and *3,000 Years Among the Microbes* can be understood as experimental works in the sense that they contribute to bringing new entities into being; they are "ontogenetic experiments" (21–22). The gradual disintegration of Des Esseintes' sensory self-control, the humanizing effect of John Wait's parasitic presence on the *Narcissus*, and Huck's *matryoshkan* relativization of species separatism all confront the readers with a view of humanity that collides with the anthropocentric and instrumental relationship to the surrounding world which dominated the Western world at the beginning of the twentieth century. In this sense, these works anticipate post-anthropocentrism.

This new view of humanity derives from a focus on the material aspects of the bacteria/body relationship. To see modernism from the point of view of bacteria is to see it in a new light because modernist criticism has traditionally been characterized by a strong cognitive focus.[7] The attention devoted to the stylistic notion of stream of consciousness is an obvious example. Georg Lukács was perhaps the first to characterize modernism as a psychological "turn inward" (Gang 117), but he inherited the idea from canonized poetological writings such as Henry James's "The Art of Fiction" (1884), Marcel Proust's *Contre Sainte-Beuve* (1896), and Virginia Woolf's "Modern Fiction" (1919). Woolf writes: "Let us record the atoms as they fall upon the mind in the order in which they fall" (161). To her, the domain of the modernist writer is "the dark places of psychology" (162). Huysmans', Conrad's, and Twain's novels invite us to take notice of the dark places of the body, as well.

Notes

1 At the same time, it is important to note that the germ theory of disease did not achieve absolute etiological dominance overnight. Competing theories were still debated in the mid-1890s.

2 For a discussion of the relationship between enchantment and modernity, see Bennett. After a discussion of three "disenchantment tales," Bennett challenges them by recalling "alternative stories about the nature of things" (84) and by pointing out "contemporary practices and experiences that are anomalous within a world understood to be wonder-disabled" (ibid.).

3 Here I refer to Margaret Mauldon's translation from 1998.

4 Mauldon translates the "nouvelles conditions d'hygiène" of the original text (Huysmans, À rebours 210) to "a different regimen of health" (Huysmans, Against Nature 174).

5 Later in the novel, this insecurity is anulled. Wait is actually ill, and he dies at sea.

6 The concern with these questions has a long theological history; see Gilhus.

7 Exceptions include Armstrong and Danius.

Works Cited

Armstrong, Tim. *Modernism, Technology, and the Body. A Cultural Study.* Cambridge: Cambridge UP, 1998.

Barnes, David S. *The Making of a Social Disease. Tuberculosis in Nineteenth-Century France.* Berkeley: The U of California P, 1995.

Bauman, Robert W. *Microbiology.* 3rd ed. Upper Saddle River: Pearson Benjamin Cummings, 2011.

Bennett, Jane. *The Enchantment of Modern Life. Attachments, Crossings, and Ethics.* Princeton: Princeton UP, 2001.

Capitan, M.L. "Microbes as Factors in Society." *Popular Science Monthly* 47(1895): 103–109.

Cassirer, Ernst. *An Essay on Man.* New Haven: Yale UP, 1945.

Connor, Steven. "CP, or a Few Don'ts by a Cultural Phenomenologist." *Parallax* 5. 2 (1999): 17–31.

Conrad, Joseph. *The Nigger of the "Narcissus".* New York: W.W. Norton and Company, 1979.

Cromie, William. "Dodging Germs." *Colliers* 23 September 1916: 33.

Danius, Sara. *The Senses of Modernism: Technology, Perception, and Modernist Aesthetics.* Ithaca: Cornell UP, 2002.

Esposito, Roberto. "Community, Immunity, Biopolitics." *Angelaki* 18. 3(2012): 83–90.

Gang, Joshua. "Mindless Modernism." *Novel: A Forum on Fiction* 46. 1(2013): 116–132.

Gilhus, Ingrid Sælid. *Animals, Gods and Humans. Changing Attitudes to Animals in Greek, Roman, and Early Christian Thought.* London: Routledge, 2006.

Hird, Myra J. *The Origins of Sociable Life: Evolution After Science Studies.* London: Palgrave Macmillan, 2009.

Huysmans, Joris-Karl. *Against Nature.* Oxford: Oxford UP, 1998.

Huysmans, Joris-Karl. *À rebours.* Paris: Au Sans Pareil, 1924.

Latour, Bruno. *The Pasteurization of France.* Cambridge: Harvard UP, 1993.

Lefebvre, Henri. *Everyday Life in the Modern World.* New York: Harper Torchbooks, 1971.

Mach, Ernst. *The Analysis of Sensations and the Relation of the Physical to the Psychical.* Chicago, IL: The Open Court Publishing Company, 1914.

Margulis, Lynn and Dorion Sagan. *Microcosmos: Four Billion Years of Evolution from Our Microbial Ancestors.* Berkeley: U of California P, 1997.

Merleau-Ponty, Maurice. *Phenomenology of Perception.* London: Routledge, 2005.

Mitchell, Robert. *Experimental Life. Vitalism in Romantic Science and Literature.* Baltimore, MD: Johns Hopkins UP, 2013.

Nietzsche, Friedrich. *Beyond Good and Evil.* Harmondsworth: Penguin Books, 1973.

Parke, Thomas Heazle. *My Personal Experiences in Equatorial Africa as Medical Officer of the Emin Pasha Relief Expedition.* London: Sampson Low, Marston and Company, 1891.

Prozorov, Sergei and Simona Rentea. *The Routledge Handbook of Biopolitics.* London: Routledge, 2017.

Söderberg, Hjalmar. *Doctor Glas.* New York: Anchor Books, 2002.

Trotter, David. "Introduction." *Cooking with Mud: The Idea of Mess in Nineteenth-Century Art and Fiction.* Oxford: Oxford UP, 2000. 1–32.

Twain, Mark. *3,000 Years Among the Microbes.* In: *Which Was the Dream and Other Symbolic Writings of the Later Years.* Berkeley: U of California P, 1968. 433–553.

Tygstrup, Frederik and Isak Winkel Holm. "Litteratur og politik." *K&K* 104(2007): 148–165.

Vigarello, Georges. *Concepts of Cleanliness: Changing Attitudes in France Since the Middle Ages.* Cambridge: Cambridge UP, 1988.

Weber, Max. "Science as a Vocation." *Max Weber's "Science as a Vocation".* Ed. Peter Lassman and Irving Velody. London: Unwin Hyman, 1989. 3–32.

Weir, David. *Decadence and the Making of Modernism.* Amherst: U of Massachusetts P, 1995.

Woolf, Virginia. "Modern Fiction." *The Essays of Virginia Woolf. Volume 4: 1925 to 1928.* London: The Hogarth Press, 1989. 157–165.

10 Being-in-Alien

The Trinity of Bodies in *Prometheus* (2012) and *Alien: Covenant* (2017)

Adnan Mahmutović and Denise Ask Nunes

Metamorphosing Bodies and the Quest for Being

The *Alien* films, the original quadrilogy (1979, 1986, 1992, 1997), featuring a female lead called Ripley, have inspired a substantial body of scholarship in gender studies, which has examined their feminine monsters, in particular the Alien queen, which, like an ant-queen, can produce hundreds of offspring (monsters). In *The Monstrous Feminine*, Barbara Creed relates Julia Kristeva's notion of the *abject* to the feminine monster as mother, which threatens that same identity it "helps to define" (9). According to Creed, the ultimate Alien monster is the parthenogenic mother (the Queen) who threatens to engulf everything she once gave birth to.[1] Thus, the Alien Queen is reduced to reproductive attributes whilst Ripley's nurturing qualities are lavished on the characters of Jonesy (from *Alien*, 1979) and Newt (from *Aliens*, 1986). Ripley becomes violent when someone threatens her adopted *baby*, as when she tells the Alien Queen, "Get away from her, you bitch." The Alien mother, in contrast is a pure monster: violent by nature, she gives birth to violence by producing perfect killers. Although human villains as corporate profiteers abound, the Alien serves as the abject Other that helps define humanity through notions such as love, compassion, companionship, and individuality-in-community.

If the original quadrilogy used the Alien metaphor to attack Capitalism's dehumanizing influences, the so-called prequels[2] *Prometheus* (2012) and *Alien: Covenant* (2017), both directed by Ridley Scott, shift this focus from the Alien to its origins and, consequently, the question of human *being*. The figure of the male android David, the precursor to all the androids in the original quadrilogy, particularly indicates this drive for origins by trying to find answers through creation itself. Since this drive involves a strong connection to the genesis of human and Alien genes, it appears to be a symbolic shift from the feminine to the masculine. The quest for origins, the quest for Being, becomes at its core tied to genetic manipulation and insemination—or masculine, versus feminine, generation.

Before the Alien Queen and her eggs came Chemical A0–3959X.91–15. The black liquid presents the masculine potential of bodily metamorphosis and original creation in contrast to the Alien womb of the hive-Queen. Scott's prequels follow what Judith Butler calls "phallic phantasy" (16), a Platonic insistence on the womb as only a receptacle for masculine creative power. Being as such becomes a seed and a sower and the feminine (womb-soil) the house of/for Being. As *Prometheus* opens, the giant, white hypermasculine engineer stands next to the waterfall, swallows the black liquid and sacrifices his body for creation; his DNA will create humanity. David is a masculine creation, Weyland's machine, created in order to find his own makers (i.e. the engineers). A third masculine creation can be seen in David's experiments. The drive to create, to change, to metamorphose, continuously positions the human among abject bodies that help define us, yet in relation to which we ourselves can be perceived as the abject that must be rejected.

In all, these scenes recall Martin Heidegger's phenomenology, which characterizes humans at their core as concerned with their *being* (*Dasein*) and a relation to *Being* (*Sein*) as such. Scott's Alien prequels ask us to rethink this relationship between beings and Being through the image of bodily interdependence. The prequels suggest that Alien and android bodies are part of this search for the human, whether in the shape of a guide (David in *Prometheus*) or a distorted humanoid monster looking back at you. Through the image of *becoming* through another being, Scott produces a rich metaphor whose meanings continuously multiply even as we try to create a firmer ground for a human being under constant violent metamorphosis. The metaphoricity is further complicated by the introduction of the android body which creates a triangular (and quite masculine) relationship as the core of what we could call a "story of Being" in these films.

In the prequels, the mysterious appearance of Aliens that can only become by growing inside another body is joined by an obsessive search for something more: Being or origin. This symbolic quest requires an actual journey into space, and on this voyage, as in any human drama, answers only bring more questions, and approaching a goal only reveals further distance to the truth. The quest itself is a series of stops on different planets, old fights, suffering, and, eventually, death. The Alien loses importance as the story of the metamorphosing Alien-man-machine trinity emerges. Being turns out to be less fixed than first believed, and this trinity exposes the vulnerable fissures in human, alien, and robot Being. As Teresa Rizzo states:

> In the *Alien* films, the human is no longer quite human. Instead, there is a mingling of Alien and human, and machine and human. The idea of the human as something pure, in a category of its own, separated clearly from other categories, is destroyed. ... in the *Alien* films the body is presented as something that is in constant process. It changes according to its environment and its encounters with other bodies.
>
> (333)

The question the *Alien* films ask is whether or not this notion of "the human as something pure" is in itself a romantic myth, always already destroyed. By evoking the myth of Prometheus, which itself was one of the sources for Heidegger's observations about Being, the films examine the potentiality for rethinking Being in terms of technology. They destroy the myth of the pure human by showing that it is something that has been introduced exactly because of the burden of that first Promethean sin, the theft/gift of *techne*.

Human, Being, and *Techne*

In the Alien prequels, the quest for Being, as Rizzo states, is strongly tied to the body, which is not the case in most religious thought or existential philosophy. The unbearable connection of Being to a trinity of bodies (human, Alien, android) makes the quest for Being a matter of *techne* or technology, whether genetic or mechanical. In Greek thought, human Being is essentially defined by technology, a means of transforming its environment and itself (its own body) and a means of understanding the truth of Being. Human beings can metamorphose by using tools, because they possess the gift of *techne* which Prometheus stole from the Gods. This is, for Heidegger, why human beings can or must be concerned with Being, while a tree cannot. What technology reveals, because it is integral to the meaning of *techne*, is the essence of human being and its connection to Being. As Heidegger explains:

> From earliest times until Plato the word *techne* is linked with the word *episteme*. Both words are names for knowing in the widest sense. They mean to be entirely at home in something, to understand and be expert in it. Such knowing provides an opening up. ... Technology is a mode of revealing. Technology comes to presence [*West*] in the realm where revealing and unconcealment take place, where *aletheia*, truth, happens.
>
> (Question Concerning Technology 13)

The *Alien* films echo the Romanticism of Mary Shelley's *Frankenstein: The Modern Prometheus* (1818), and its warnings against the dangers of technology now inherent to science fiction. However, if Shelley tried to liberate humans from the burden (or the original sin) of *techne*, the *Alien* prequels show how humans are always already technological. Technology, or as it is called in the films, engineering, is the origin and destiny of humanity. Already engineered, humans become engineers themselves who can transform the world, their bodies, and even create in their own image. What is most terrifying, perhaps, is not so much the monsters as what their abject bodies reveal to us about our own being. Heidegger writes: "What is dangerous is not technology. ... The essence of technology, as a destining of revealing, is the danger" (Question Concerning Technology 28).

The opening of *Alien: Covenant* establishes a drive for knowledge about origins as well as a first human perspective on creation. In the time of the original movies, the drive for profit trumps the drive for knowledge. Despite this, Tony Safford identifies the android Ash's scientific impulse as a "pure quest for knowledge" that "results in evil" (Byars et al. 297). There can be no pure quest because of the profit seeking impetus at the core of this drive. This selfish drive can be seen in the prequels as well in relation to Weyland, yet David is driven by a purer desire to understand creation. Weyland observes to David:

WEYLAND: "I am your father ... ambulate ... [watches the android walk] ... perfect."
DAVID: "Am I?"
WEYLAND: "Perfect?"
DAVID: "Your son?"
WEYLAND: "You are my creation ... what is your name?"
DAVID: "David"
...
DAVID: "If you created me? Who created you?"
WEYLAND: "The question of the ages. Which I hope you and I will answer one day."
...
DAVID: "You seek your creator and I am looking at mine. I will serve you and yet you are human. You will die, I will not."
WEYLAND: "Bring me the tea, David."

This scene establishes central thematic threads: perfection, the relationship between creator and creation, and, most importantly the hierarchy between them. Already, although the quest is yet to begin, we discern the answers: the android is too human to be perfect; there is a lack of intimacy between creator and creation; and the creation will supersede the creator. It is through Weyland's creation that he intends to find his own origins; as Heidegger argued, technology provides the hope of revelation. Weyland has spent his entire lifetime contemplating his origin, purpose, and destiny. He believes that meeting his maker will answer all of his questions.

Prometheus expands on this idea. When the crew of USCSS Prometheus wake from cryo sleep, Weyland's hologram tells them that the android David is the closest thing Weyland will ever have to a son, but he is not human. David will never grow old and never die, yet he is unable to appreciate this fact because he does not have a soul. Weyland makes the distance between maker and creation explicit in this scene and it is in this vein that David later indicates that meeting one's maker might therefore not be the cathartic experience Weyland, as well as, for example, Shaw and Holloway, hoped for. David asks Holloway why the humans created him:

HOLLOWAY: "We made you because we could."
DAVID: "Can you imagine how disappointing it would be for you to hear the same thing from your creator? May I ask you something, how far would you go to get what you came all this way for, your answers? What would you be willing to do?"

HOLLOWAY: "Anything and everything."

David then puts a drop of black liquid (Chemical A0–3959X.91–15) into Holloway's drink. Searching for answers through creation, David uses the black liquid to inseminate Holloway who in turn inseminates Elisabeth Shaw with a squid-like monster she later aborts. The quest for origins might be believed to bring one closer to one's being, but David shows that getting answers might be a matter of creation through metamorphosis. It is not our maker that defines us; we become through the abject bodies that we create. David and Holloway's interaction indicates that the discovery of the giant engineers does not solve the riddle but only raises further questions.

What is important here is the notion that an object produced through technology, the android, too, can embody a concern with Being. In *Alien: Covenant*, for example, Walter says that he was "designed to supersede every earlier model, but ...," and David adds "you were not allowed to create." Androids like David are often virtual zealots and his pursuit of origins drives him to commit genocide of the so-called engineers. Like humans, they are given the gift of technology and become, like humans, the destroyers of their own creators. The gift of *techne* becomes a *de facto* weapon against the creator(s) and this destructive impulse is at the core of creation.

Death as a Precondition for Creation

In *Prometheus*'s initial scene, the engineer dissolves his own body to fertilize planet earth with his cells, demonstrating the close connection between creation and destruction. As David says, "sometimes to create, one must first destroy." Destruction is a precondition for creation and the drive to kill one's maker is a strong impetus in this process of metamorphosis. Just as God created humans in his own image, the same can be said for the engineers and Weyland. The image of the engineers in humanity goes DNA-deep, while David is crafted to look like a human.[3] Drawing on Creed's observation, "The subject who fantasizes about giving birth to himself does so in order to cut his tie to the mother" (48), it is, in a way, an attempt at a purely masculine creative force. One could also say that Weyland's creation of David unknowingly separates him from his origins, even though he seeks to find them. This separation is later violently literalized when David bombards the engineers (Weyland's creators) with the black liquid (Chemical A0–3959X.91–15). This scene hints at the dangers of uncontrolled metamorphosis. Instead of changing and thereby understanding one's Being, the engineers' bodies are dissolved. The danger of the revelatory power of *techne* is the fine line between Being and destruction. Metamorphosis can bring us closer to Being but it might just as well destroy us.

In the Alien prequels, understanding one's Being through separation is always a form of technological operation. David's creation of the Aliens is a particularly clear example of this separation. If we return to the scene where Weyland calls David "perfect," there is already an attempt to distinguish himself from his imperfect maker. Firstly, a hierarchical inversion means that the human is now the abject that must be destroyed, and secondly, David uses technology to create something perfect—the Alien. The quest for origins, then, is a series of separations from those who participated in one's creation. The quest is therefore a shedding or destruction of one's origin, or that which attempts to define, and thereby limit, one's possibility to be, or Being. The crux here is that this quest is always already a failure because it envisions Being or origin as the end point, something ideal one can find deep in space (like the journey to find the engineers on their planet). Creation through metamorphosis is embodied which is why there can be no ultimate origin, there was a body before and there will be one after.

Technology is, in other words, not detached from the body. In *Alien: Covenant* it is clear that David is the creator of the Aliens we recognize from the original movies. However, the body of Elisabeth Shaw was not enough to create the perfect monster, and David's work suffered because it lacked one "essential ingredient." He needs real human bodies to create. The death of his makers not only frees him to create, but ironically, they become the very soil for his creative force.

The monster, then, is a co-creation between the human body and technological manipulation. In "Human Artifice and the Science Fiction Film," J.P. Telotte argues that there is a "dangerous and even self-destructive impulse behind that fascination with the power of science or some select knowledge to enable man to duplicate himself artificially. This Faustian impulse, however, typically tries to go masked as a Promethean one" (45). Monsters are the result of such an imperfect duplication (Stacey 252), which is probably why the creator many time seeks to destroy its creation as well. In the earlier movies, there was no sign of this "original creation." Monsters generated monsters. The prequels reveal that this pattern was created by a being neither human nor Alien, a third thing. The mysterious black liquid of pure creation, as seed, is the governing metaphor that represents depersonalized masculine creation as pure technology, which, ironically, makes creation highly personal because their engineering metamorphoses the body. Equally ironically, the one who succeeds in creating this perfection is a machine. Hence, the triad of bodies—human, Alien, android—are tied through their likenesses and differences, natural, technological, and symbolic.[4] The trinity of bodies indicates a constant struggle with the double that never brings them home, but only further and further out into space. This returns to the initial comment that this is where the abject can metamorphose and challenge Being which in the end helps bring us closer to it. However, because *techne* is at the core of our being, continuous metamorphosis and creation will never settle Being, but only challenge it.

Lack at the Core

The myth of Prometheus suggests that the gift of *techne* was given to replace something essential missing at the core of human beings, something connected to Being, to the creative power, to something that matters. In the Alien prequels, the human–robot binary was dismantled through the very *techne* intended to distinguish human beings from objects and simultaneously allow them access to Being. Yet the Alien brings in another relation, that between the human and the animal. We thus enter a Derridean realm of unsustainable binaries.

The Alien is described in animalistic or insect-like terms, acting on pure (killing) instinct, through a hive-Queen whose purpose is to multiply and who must be terminated for the species to die. Each opposition: human/animal (Alien), human/machine (android), and animal (Alien)/machine (android) identify semantic interrelations and ontological hierarchies. In *The Animal That Therefore I Am*, Derrida argues that "when tradition defines the human ... as *rational animal* ... it has always in fact opposed us to all the rest of animalkind ... conversely, to define the animal, in an essentially negative way, as deprived of whatever is presumed to be 'proper' to the human" (x). A *lack* is thus what most clearly defines both animal and machine in a lower hierarchical relation to humans. In the animal/machine binary, a clear nature/culture divide privileges culture. A hierarchy is thus unavoidable in these juxtapositions but it is somewhat detached from reality.

Despite this, Derrida asks whether humanity can only be defined by this other who *lacks*. To a certain extent this is the case, as in "I am what I am not." However, when human/animal/machine are merged and interact in *Prometheus* and *Alien: Covenant*, the preordained hierarchical structure crumbles. Bojan Žikić examines how the Alien-as-hive functions as the opposite identity marker in comparison with humans, lacking free will and morality (115). Humanity should come out on top, having all the properties that the Alien lacks; however, in this case, the Alien, with its complete lack of morality, is actually perfect and above humans.

In *Alien*, the Company is well aware of the nature of the xenomorph and Ash is meant to ensure its return to earth. Ash speaks of its purity with admiration, an opinion that can only be preprogrammed, thus, echoing the Company's view. He mockingly tells the survivors on *Nostromo* that the Alien is perfect. "Its structural perfection is matched only by its hostility. ... A survivor, unclouded by conscience, remorse, or delusions of morality." David echoes this view in *Alien: Covenant* when he tells Walter that "I've found perfection. I've created it." There is thus a hierarchical inversion between machine and animal, which spills into the human. The Machine created perfection, the Animal, and humanity becomes a late-night snack to an Alien that should be hierarchically lower than them both. Nevertheless, Derrida provides a model for contradictory treatment of animals in human discourse as embodying "absolute goodness, absolute innocence, prior to good and evil ... without fault and defect (that would be its superiority or inferiority), but also the animal as absolute evil, cruelty, murderous savagery" (64). The ability to be superior "like this," makes it inferior. In other words, the alien's perfection stops it from superseding the human but in this move towards the top, human frailty is displayed. Even though the binary holds, it has become more vulnerable. Additionally, David's lack of morality makes him a superior creator and allows him to strive for perfection. Morality hinders purity and creation, even as it is held to be the highest human standard. Human is superseded in creative capacity and survival by animal and machine, but morality, a weakness, still supposedly supports our superior position. However, it has now, to a certain extent, been identified as a lack. Morality is just one example that shows how the hierarchy, and hence Being, is continuously rearranged amongst the trinity.

Human beings find a lack at their very core, a lack that is manifested by a concern for their own being, their origin, their place in the universe. This is why there is a simultaneous desire for origins and creation. But this lack is present in the android and in the Alien creature. They all need something and are willing to go to any lengths to acquire it. They all kill and exploit. There is no point of rest, for the lack is essential to them all. It may appear that android and animal/Alien exist as abject entities that define the Being of human beings. But it is impossible to maintain hierarchies exactly because all three have something in common, *techne*. *Techne* in the animal/Alien is produced through technology (genetic engineering), and ultimately what defines the Alien is the ability to create itself by manipulating its own features through access to the genetic material of its host. In fact, the Alien thus becomes the perfect embodiment of *techne*, used without conscious thought, without intention, mechanically and following genetic programing. The purity that both Ash and David see in the Alien is the ultimate ability to metamorphose. This metamorphosis seems to be entirely organic and therefore not technological but is later revealed to be nothing but technological. It presents the highest form of engineering, a self-sustainable technology. In some sense, one could argue that the Alien engineers itself by processing the DNA of the host body, which is not merely an environment to grow in. On the contrary, the Alien engineers the host's DNA and extracts that which is absolutely best and use it for its own metamorphosis. This is why the android is fascinated by the creature that, as the ultimate product of engineering, is the purest form, metaphorically speaking, of the idea that Being is *techne*, but not just as the endless possibility for transformation. In other words, Being is not a constant or unchangeable, unless we see it as a principle of transformation.

Conclusion

The android figure ultimately distinguishes the Alien films from stories, like Prometheus or *Frankenstein*, concerning the combination of the topics of genesis and technology. The myth of Prometheus is a warning, and *Frankenstein* begins to illustrate how practically every popular story about the relationship between technical ingenuity and human being is a horror story. The Matrix trilogy, the Terminator franchise, the Blade Runner films, like much other serious science fiction shows, again and again, how technologically created beings become murderous agents. The latest development in the Alien franchise goes a step further, staging a search for Being which is at its purest also genocidal. The Alien prequels distill this search as Being-in-technology, technology-in-Being, and ultimately Being-in-Alien. Endless engineering does not lead to closure, where the characters find something akin to a soul or God. What is always already present is the notion that Being as such is always already technological and embodied, exactly the way the android is entirely a machine and entirely human as well (and neither-nor), exactly the way the Alien is both animal and human. The trinity of bodies in these films, which are both essentially different and essentially the same, moves us far from the notion of technology-as-tools as in the Prometheus myth. Rather technology is only suggestive of the embodiment of *techne* in all three beings. This *techne* is shown through constant desire to fill a lack and a need to transform.

In the Alien films, then, metamorphosis through technology does not have an end, and despite the strong focus on origins, it does not really have a beginning. It is important for the characters and of course the audience to see beyond the science fiction universe to the wider notion of *techne* and how it reveals something about the Being of human beings, as Heidegger suggests (Being and Time 14). Since his definition of Being takes the shape of zealots, genocidal androids, and alien monsters—that is, nothing even remotely positive—we see over and again a fundamental fear of Being, which Heidegger only marginally addressed when speaking of the notion of danger. Being is terrifying. It is abject like the bodies that represent it metaphorically. It is ultimately fascinating and ultimately terrifying because it is close and yet ultimately alien. The terror of/in Being is not mysterious, though the prequels show how humans want to make it mysterious, a matter of some eternal quest. Being reveals itself exactly through the endless repetition of generic tropes that were probably best portrayed by Shelley. The fear of technology in genre fiction is the fear of that which defines Being, and therefore also human "being," *techne*. As such it is like the fear of original sin. The theft/gift of *techne* is a burden exactly because it is at the same time an inherent part of our being and also not truly ours. It reminds us, through the alien the android bodies, that we too are abject.

Notes

1 Also see Stephen Scobie's "What's the Story, Mother?: The Mourning of the Alien" and Lynda Zwinger's "Blood Relations: Feminist Theory Meets the Uncanny Bug Mother."
2 The notion of "prequel" in the movie industry signifies stories belonging to a franchise but set chronologically before the original stories.
3 There are indeed attempts to point out distinctions. The male android is supposed to be as far from nature as he can be, which is shown in the scene in *Alien: Covenant* where he forces himself on Daniels and kisses her only to ask "Is this how it's done?" This scene can be compared to the scene in *Prometheus* where Vickers is asked by the flirting captain whether she is a robot and she answers "My room. 10 minutes." Intimacy and sex become proof of one's humanity; the scene also shows how denigrating it was for Vickers to be mistaken for a robot. She seems to establish her humanity through an avowal of the abject.

4 Creed argues: "The fully symbolic body must bear no indication of its debt to nature. In Kristeva's view the image of woman's body, because of its maternal functions, acknowledges its 'debt to nature' and consequently is more likely to signify the abject" (11).

Works Cited

Bundtzen, Lynda K. "Monstrous Mothers: Medusa, Grendel, and Now Alien." *Film Quarterly* 40. 3(1987): 11–17.

Butler, Judith. *Bodies That Matter*. London: Routledge, 2011.

Byars, Jackie, Jeff Gould, Peter Fitting, Judith Newton, Tony Safford, and Clayton Lee. "Symposium on *Alien*." *Science Fiction Studies* 7. 3(1980): 278–304.

Cameron, James, dir. *Aliens*. United States: 20th Century Fox, 1986.

Creed, Barbara. *The Monstrous Feminine: Film, Feminism, Psychoanalysis*. London: Routledge, 1993.

Derrida, Jacques. *The Animal That Therefore I Am*. Trans. David Willis. New York: Fordham UP, 2008.

Heidegger, Martin. *Being and Time: A Translation of Sein und Zeit*. Trans. Joan Stambaugh. New York: SUNY Press, 1996.

Heidegger, Martin. *The Question Concerning Technology*. Trans. William Lovitt. New York: Harper and Row, 1993.

Rizzo, Teresa. "The Alien Series: A Deleuzian Perspective." *Women: A Cultural Review* 15. 3(2004): 330–344.

Scobie, Stephen. "What's the Story, Mother?: The Mourning of the Alien." *Science Fiction Studies* 20. 1(1993): 80–93.

Scott, Ridley, dir. *Alien*. United States: 20th Century Fox, 1979.

Scott, Ridley, dir. *Alien: Covenant*. United States: 20th Century Fox, 2017.

Scott, Ridley, dir. *Prometheus*. United States: 20th Century Fox, 2012.

Stacey, Jackie. "She is Not Herself: The Deviant Relations of *Alien Resurrection*." *Screen* 44. 3(2003): 251–276.

Telotte, J.P. "Human Artifice and the Science Fiction Film." *Film Quarterly* 36. 3(1983): 44–51.

Žikić, Bojan. "We are Me, and They are Hive. Individual and Collective Identity as Relational Characteristic of Humans and Aliens in Science Fiction." *Antropologija* 10. 1(2010): 111–122.

Zwinger, Lynda. "Blood Relations: Feminist Theory Meets the Uncanny Bug Mother." *Hypatia* 7. 2(1992): 74–90.

Part III

Aging, Decline, and Death

11 Embodied Transitions in Michel de Montaigne

Nora Martin Peterson and Peter Martin

How does the mind–body relationship develop over the human life span? What role does embodiment play in the transition to later life? And what might we learn about cognition and mortality from looking at essays from the sixteenth century? Embodied cognition has become an important part of the psychological and gerontological literature. During the last decade, psychologists and gerontologists have begun to use embodied cognition as a theoretical framework and to investigate how cognitive functions are intertwined with the body and with physical actions, particularly as the body changes over time. M.C. Costello and E.K. Bloesch define embodied cognition as "a theoretical framework which posits that cognitive function is intimately intertwined with the body and physical actions" (1). The major premise of this approach is that body and mind are closely linked (Foglia and Wilson). Whereas cognitive theory views cognitive processes as the "center" of all behaviors and perceptions, and the body is an independent vehicle for the execution of behavior, embodied cognition emphasizes the direct interrelatedness of body and cognition highlighting that the body is a "co-producer" of cognitive processes (Costello and Bloesch).

During his life, Michel de Montaigne (1533–1592) served as the mayor of Bordeaux and as a religious and political negotiator, but he is best known for his collection of *Essays*. Written in the sixteenth century, these essays, which were literary in nature and which can be broadly described as reflections on various subjects from negotiating a peace treaty, to the relationship between fathers and sons, to the role of the imagination, might seem like an unlikely place to start looking for evidence of embodied cognition. But Montaigne professes a deep interest in reflecting on what we would today call embodiment. "I am myself the matter of my book" (3), he proclaims in his preface to the reader, and throughout the *Essays*, which are by various turns full of humor, circular logic, self-assessment, and perhaps above all, open-endedness, readers are introduced to a man who accepts, takes advantage of, and is curious to explore the interrelatedness of the mind and the body. Montaigne published several editions of the *Essays* between the first (in 1580) and the last (published posthumously in 1588) and in each edition, he revised, added on to, or even reversed his opinions from previous versions. He reveals interest not only in embodying himself textually, but also in exploring an active cognitive practice of self-embodiment. Indeed, Montaigne appears to embrace the "unstable relationship between himself and his text" (Claus 21). Just as humans have an ever changing, at times unstable, but always necessary relationship with their bodies, Montaigne demonstrates that the same can be true of a relationship between writer and text.

Literary scholarship on Montaigne is vast; as are studies that explore how Montaigne's embodiment is informative to the way we read him.[1] Relatedly, others have explored how Montaigne's writing itself is a documentation of his body: writing as textual embodiment of the self, an "uncertain bodily odyssey" (O'Neill 74).[2] But fewer studies have focused on what we, twenty-first century readers and scholars, can learn from Montaigne's embodied methodology in an interdisciplinary context. This approach requires creating active links between literary texts and other disciplines such as gerontology.[3] The field of cognition has, increasingly, been emerging as a fruitful angle from which to look at literature. Literary and cultural studies explore ways in which literature creates, participates in, and reflects the human experience. Scholars of this discipline are deeply interested in ways in which text and human experience interact. By their very nature, the questions raised by literary scholars often share methods of inquiry with a variety of other disciplines. Terence Cave recently suggested that the study of literature is essentially a "cognitive discipline" (12) because of the way it "makes things happen, gives a local habitation and a name to unfamiliar feelings and events, or makes familiar ones strange" (1). Gerontology as a discipline provides a perspective of physical, functional, and cognitive changes experienced by individuals over time and how these changes fit within the framework of successful aging (Martin et al.).

Reading through the lenses of embodiment, health, and geropsychology, we will consider Montaigne's relationship to his body, mind, and text from a cognitive perspective.[4] Montaigne writes about a variety of embodied transitions: a near-death experience, aging and cognitive decline, and a lengthy discussion of how to face one's own mortality. In the following pages we will focus on a few of these embodied transitions. We will highlight moments in which Montaigne's body—through his text—documents the aging process and the passage of time (Yandell 78–81). And we will suggest that Montaigne's text mirrors human transitions throughout life.

By constructing a textual building whose architecture remains constantly in progress, Montaigne creates a parallel between his text and cognitive embodiment over the human life span. Thus, we believe, looking to Montaigne opens up new ways to explore current and future work on the mind–body relationship and on successful aging. Both in terms of what he writes and how he writes it, Montaigne shows readers that the transition through life is an embodied one, and that accepting the body as "co-producer" of cognitive processes (Costello and Bloesch 267) can lead to a more balanced acceptance of the complexity that accompanies the aging process and how we view older people. We hope to show that Montaigne's essays—innovative in their own time—remain important in discussing embodied transitions today.

Montaigne and the Mind–Body Relationship

> Men do not know the natural *infirmity* of their mind: it does nothing but *ferret* and *quest*, and keeps incessantly *whirling around*, building up and *becoming entangled* in its own work, like our silkworms, and is *suffocated* in it ... It thinks it notices from a distance some sort of glimmer of imaginary light and truth; but while *running* toward it, it is crossed by so many new quests, that it *strays* from the road, bewildered.
>
> (Montaigne III.13, 817; emphasis added)

In this passage from "Of Experience," the last essay in Montaigne's collection, the author uses bodily vocabulary to describe the inner workings of the mind. Running, entanglement, and suffocation, are a few of the words Montaigne chooses to highlight the mind's natural weakness. It is worth noting that the French title, "De l'Experience," is derived from "faire l'essai de" in sixteenth-century French. This roughly translates to "to try out," or "to experience" [for the first time]. But it is also worth noting the proximity of "faire l'essai de" and Montaigne's own *Essays* ("essais" in French): they, too, are something to work through, try out, sample. Thus, an experience is, by its very definition, both bodily and something to be reflected on. An experience is a transition from one moment, or thought, or state of being, to another. Because we inevitably participate in the moments and thoughts of our own lives, experiences are implicitly embodied, involving both our bodies and our minds. Montaigne is explicit about this connection, and insists on the inextricability of one from the other. The same kind of corporal emphasis exists in many other passages of the *Essays*; indeed, Montaigne often relies on the body's vocabulary when he describes transitional states, such as the cognitive decline that frequently accompanies old age (Yandell 78). In "Of Physiognomy," for example, he suggests that the mind "grows constipated and sluggish as it grows old" (III.12, 809). His thoughts, and his thoughts about how these thoughts change during the aging process, are marked by traces of the body.

Montaigne's writing about the human life span reflects the common thinking of his time. He mentions, at various points, historical examples of the ideal age at retirement (I.57, 237), the development of the intellectual soul (I.57, 237–238), and the customary life expectancy, which he mentions having exceeded (I.57, 237). But he also acknowledges the tension that develops between the mind and the body during the aging process (Yandell 78):

> In my youth I needed to warn and urge myself to stick to my duty: blitheness and health do not go so well, they say, with these wise and serious reflections. At present I am in another state. The conditions of old age warn me, sober me, and preach to me only too much. ... This body of mine flees disorder and fears it. It is my body's turn to guide my mind toward reform.
>
> (III.5, 638)

When Montaigne reflects on the differences between young and old people, he grants advantages to both. While the young are healthy and agile, older individuals are wise and serious. The body's dominance transitions into a dominance of the mind in later years. This transition corresponds to many of the personal characteristics discussed in research on aging: as people get older, they often become more reflective and introverted ("the conditions of old age warn me"), as well as more conscientious ("this body of mine flees disorder") (Srivastava et al.). Changes in vision, hearing, and mobility also may start in midlife and often continue on a downward trajectory throughout the second half of life (Tinetti).

From the gerontological perspective, wisdom may well be the end result of identity development. In Erik Erikson's (1959) theory of development, wisdom is attained with the resolution of the eighth and final stage of life: the last developmental task is to cognitively "integrate" previous experiences and one's life as it has been. Integrity is a focus on priorities of the self (Staudinger and Glück) and results in wisdom. For Montaigne, the advantage to this loss of physical prowess is that in old age, people are afforded "more freedom to prate and more indiscretion in talking about oneself" (III.2, 611). During the transition to older age, humans realize the strength and wisdom of their mind as their physical strength and health begins to decline.

But Montaigne notes that the transition to a superiority of mind is not always a straightforward transfer. Often, it is complicated by cognitive decline. Naturally, this would be something to fear, since it would disrupt the already fragile and arguable advantage of the mind over the body in older age. In the passage above, Montaigne emphasizes that he fears and flees from "disorder."[5] In other essays he is similarly frank about the negative effects of cognitive decline on older adults. Indeed, physical changes are often accompanied by cognitive changes in later life. In some (but certainly not all) older adults, these changes result in cognitive disorders, such as Alzheimer's disease or other dementias, but in most older adults changes are gradual, and they do not limit everyday functioning. These "usual" changes may affect short-term ("working") memory (Zacks), processing speed (Salthouse), and spatial abilities (Klencklen, Després, and Dufour). More recently, cognitive changes have also been linked to physical activity levels (Kraft). Even though Montaigne establishes a binary between cognitive and physical decline, he himself questions this opposition when he repeatedly writes about cognitive decline in embodied terms (Yandell 81). In "Of Repentance" he writes that "old age puts more wrinkles in our minds than on our faces; and we never, or rarely, see a soul that in growing old does not come to smell sour and musty" (III.2, 620). Souls can smell musty just as little as minds can be wrinkled, and for Montaigne, the two go hand in hand.

Even Montaigne's anxieties about cognitive decline are expressed using the vocabulary of the body. The interplay between cognitive and physical function has been noted by life span developmental psychologist Paul Baltes, who reflects on the "incomplete architecture of human ontogeny." Baltes suggests that because of evolutionary selection pressures, biological potential decreases ("physical decline") but is compensated by a greater need for culture ("cognitive growth") with age. Because of the increasing imbalance of growth relative to decline, the life span architecture may become more incomplete with age. In Baltes' view, the increasing decline in functioning relative to the potential for growth requires individuals to direct more psychological and social resources toward the regulation and management of loss.

Baltes' view, however, stands in contrast to alternative gerontological perspectives that emphasize the potential for successful aging well into very late life. In their seminal paper on successful aging, Rowe and Kahn emphasize that aging will be "successful" or "optimal" if aging individuals avoid disease and disability, and function well physically and cognitively.[6] Physical health, cognitive health, and social engagement are all important aspects of successful aging. The arguments put forth by Baltes, on the one hand, and Rowe and Kahn, on the other, need not be mutually exclusive. Incompletion does not preclude success; indeed, Montaigne seems to suggest that evolution, contradiction, and (self) revision are important components to life. Recognizing this seems to be a key part of the way that Montaigne embodies himself, even when he is writing about the transition to a chapter of life that is understandably filled with uncertainty.

Whether it is viewed as an incomplete architecture or as successful aging, the last chapter of life may be viewed with fear, and there is fear, and social stigma surrounding cognitive decline in Montaigne's works. Readers get the sense that cognitive loss can be equated with loss of control over one's own departure from life. If the process happens quietly, slowly, unremarkably, then embodied cognition remains intact for longer periods of time. Montaigne writes that "God is merciful to those whose life he takes away bit by bit; that is the only benefit of old age. ... Thus do I melt and slip away from myself" (III.13, 845). But on the other hand, if cognition—meant to be at a greater advantage in older age than the body's physical loss of strength—begins to decline prematurely, then the natural transition into old age becomes something to be feared: "How stupid it would be of my mind if it were to feel the last leap of this decline, which is already so far advanced, as acutely as if it were the whole fall. I hope this will not happen" (III.13, 845). In another passage, he writes: "What strange metamorphoses I see old age producing every day in many of my acquaintances! It is a powerful malady, and it creeps up on us naturally and imperceptibly. We need a great provision of study, and great precaution, to avoid the imperfections it loads upon us, or at least to slow up their progress" (III.2, 620–621). This transition is one in which mind and body are once again in a mutually dependent relationship. The body is necessary to describe cognition, while cognition is necessary to stay in control and take stock of one's physical losses.

Montaigne is frank about acknowledging the obstacles faced by many who lose their cognitive faculties before their bodies grow weak: "Sometimes it is the body that first surrenders to age, sometimes, too, it is the mind; and I have seen enough whose brains were enfeebled before their stomach and legs; and inasmuch as this is a malady hardly perceptible to the sufferer and obscure in its symptoms, it is all the more dangerous" (I.57, 238). Again, Montaigne implies that cognitive decline is more problematic than physical aging because the former undermines the supposed advantage that people gain in older life. It would seem that there is a tipping point at which cognitive embodiment is no longer a symbiotic relationship. Thus, rather than declare the victory of mind over body, or of the atrophy of the human mind *and* body as the only possible outcomes during the aging process, Montaigne suggests that mind and body are in a constantly evolving transition, always adapting to whatever relationship needs to be built up given the circumstances.

Cynthia Skenazi notes that our attitudes towards age and aging are not so different from those of the early modern period. Montaigne, for example, refuses to see aging as unproblematic, and his text highlights "the complexities of aging as a cultural and psychological notion" (580). Indeed, many of the same complexities exist today in discussions about how to define successful aging (Peterson and Martin). What we can learn from Montaigne is that discord and ambivalence are part of the human aging process. Montaigne's writing invites, even depends upon, incompleteness and at the same time, it contains within it a constant sense that his mind and his body accompany him textually along his journey. Is this so different from the many kinds of transitions that humans face over the course of a life span?

Montaigne on the Transition from Life to Death

Now that we have considered the mutually dependent relationship of the mind and the body as they transition into older age, and have established the omnipresence of bodily vocabulary in Montaigne's thoughts about cognitive decline, we will turn to ways in which embodied cognition can help aging individuals prepare for and come to peace with their own mortality. This transition, also referred to in the gerontological literature as "gerotranscendence," challenges older adults to reflect on their own experiences and on ways in which to cope with loss (Tornstam). Here, too, the transition from living to dying appears to be one that calls for practice (even though, as Montaigne points out, practicing death is, in practical terms, impossible), and one that equally involves the mind and the body. And again, Montaigne seems to experiment with the relationship between the two in his own embodiment of the transition. The most powerful of commentaries about facing one's own mortality comes in an essay called "On Practice."

In this essay, Montaigne remembers a day when, during a journey home, he is thrown from his horse. He loses consciousness, even calls himself "dead," for a span of over two hours. No one is able to revive him. In today's terms, Montaigne's account would be commonly recognizable as a "near-death experience." These experiences might include impressions of being "outside one's own physical body" and/or "visions of deceased relatives with a general transcendence of spatial and temporal boundaries" (Greyson). Montaigne writes:

Those who were with me, after having tried all the means they could to bring me round, thinking me dead, took me in their arms and were carrying me with great difficulty to my house. ... On the way, and after I had been taken for dead for more than two full hours, I began to move and breathe.

(II.6, 269)

Montaigne's physical death is accompanied by cognitive absence—he cannot write, think, or speak during this period. But in projecting himself back into the space of physical death in this essay, he reconstructs the experience. Specifically, Montaigne reflects on the relative peace he experiences cognitively even while his body is in the throes of a physically distressing event. He writes:

It seemed to me that my life was hanging only by the tip of my lips; I closed my eyes in order, it seemed to me, to help push it out, and took pleasure in growing languid and letting myself go. It was an idea that was only floating on the surface of my soul, as delicate and feeble as all the rest, but in truth not only free from distress but mingled with that sweet feeling that people who have let themselves slide into sleep.

(II.6, 269–270)

Here, Montaigne uses embodied language in order to describe his cognitive state: his life is hanging by the tip of his lips, he closes his eyes, he pushes life out, lets it go. This unusually vivid image (which is the same in the original French) directly links the body to death; life lingers, hanging onto the lips (a part of the body that links the interior to the exterior), as if to imply that whether he will live or die depends on his soul's embodied hesitation between existence and nonexistence. At the same time, he lingers over the sweetness of the *disembodiment* of the experience. Rather than feel the physical pain of the fall, he is able to drift easily in and out of consciousness. Because he believes that he is approaching death, he tries to make the transition as easy and painless as possible. He comments on the fact that his thoughts take place in an abstract, a purportedly disembodied space: "These were idle thoughts, in the clouds, set in motion by the sensations of the eyes and ears; they did not come from within me. I did not know, for all that, where I was coming from or where I was going, nor could I weigh and consider what I was asked ... I was not there at all" (II.6, 271). A sense of peace and painlessness as well as a sense of removal from the world is often characterized by people who recall their near-death experience (Mauro). The declaration that Montaigne "was not there at all" appears at first glance to dissolve into an existential contradiction: how can a physical subject "not be there"? The moment suggests a distancing of cognition from the body, a dissolution of the very relationship of dependence that Montaigne and today's scholarship insist upon. But perhaps there is more at stake here. First of all, in this moment, Montaigne's cognition takes over, numbing what would otherwise be an unbearably painful embodied experience, especially in the age before anesthetics. But the ability to withstand such physical pain depends on the mind's ability to block it. In this way, cognitive embodiment in Montaigne's near-death moment actually proves the mutual dependency between mind and body. And indeed, Montaigne adds that "when I came back to life and regained my powers, ... which was two or three hours later, I felt myself all of a sudden caught up again in the pains" (II.6, 272). His mind's temporary ability to numb the worst of the pain allows his body to heal to the point that he will survive—physically and mentally.

What about those who do not, or will not survive? All of us, Montaigne is well aware, will at some point be dealt a mortal blow or succumb to old age and, finally, to death. Montaigne uses his near-death experience as a kind of case study, an example for how actual death might feel for people. And Montaigne suggests that though we might see their bodies in a state that appears to be painful, this might not be the case at all, and that a similar kind of separation might be occurring internally:

> I believe that this is the same in which people find themselves whom we see fainting with weakness in the agony of death; and I maintain that we pity them without cause, supposing that they are agitated by grievous pains or have their soul oppressed by painful thought.
>
> (II.6, 269–270)

What people fear, Montaigne writes, stems from the anticipation of death, from the unknown, from something that one cannot practice before it happens. Gerontological studies suggest that fear of death is actually greater among younger adults and declines with increasing age, particularly after the age of 60 (Cicirelli).[7] For the oldest-old population, qualitative interviews suggests that this age group is not likely to fear death itself; instead, they fear the dying process (Johnson and Barer). By textually embodying a transition that fills many people with as much fear today as it did five hundred years ago, Montaigne provides some comfort for those wondering what it will feel like, for those fearing the pain that they imagine when they see a loved one on their death bed. Montaigne hopes to change the cultural representation of death. His strategy, sharing a moment that for him was the example of cognitive embodiment at its best, is to offer an alternative to those who expect the opposite.

At the moment before death, Montaigne suggests that the mind and body are working together most closely. It is the pinnacle of a lifetime of work together: the mind can overcome the pain of the body and allow the individual to slip out of life. Achieving this sort of peaceful transition out of one's embodiment comes after years of "listening to his body" (O'Neill 215), of knowing himself, of coming to an embodied understanding of the need to die. In the end, Montaigne's focus on bodily pain and the cognitive representation of death allows him to accept finitude. When decline of health is not deniable any more, when death is inevitable, acceptance becomes the last stage of the dying process (Kübler-Ross). This kind of perspective, which traces the relationship of body and mind through the transition to old age and towards death, shows cognitive embodiment at its best. It also highlights that the mutual dependence of mind and body can be a symbiotic one, even during the last and hardest of transitions.

The point, perhaps, is that the relationship into which mind and body enter at birth has developed, by late in the human life span, into something so finely tuned, so symbiotically matched, that we do not even recognize how well it is functioning. Just when it would seem that cognitive embodiment would fail is when it is at its best. Throughout his *Essays*, Montaigne shows an interest in highlighting moments of complexity and ambivalence in the human experience. Above all, Montaigne insists that while complexity and ambivalence are inevitable parts of life, we also have an invaluable tool at our disposal for the hardest transitions that we as humans will face. By recognizing and embracing the constant interplay between mind and body at work within ourselves, Montaigne suggests, we can quite literally change the way in which we think about embodied transitions. Rather than being condemned to face with fear what culture often depicts as the weakness and atrophy that come with old age, we can cognitively accept the things that we do not know. Successful aging, for Montaigne, is the acceptance of the transition from mind to body, and of the increasing role that cognitive embodiment can play later in life. In the twenty-first century as in the sixteenth, embodied transitions are made richer when we see the revisions, contradictions, and hesitations that accompany them as complementary rather than conflicting.

Notes

1 See, for example, O'Sullivan; Cave; Yandell; and O'Neill. For a general overview, see Thane.
2 For a seminal work on Montaigne's embodied movement throughout the *Essays*, see Starobinski.
3 Cave suggests that the reason why cognitive readings are not popular in literary studies partly lies in the dominance of other interpretive frameworks (Saussurean structuralism, deconstruction, postcolonialism, etc.)—frameworks that depend more on binaries, and the undoing thereof, than on symbiotic relationships such as the one Cave proposes between literature and cognition (15).
4 Among the few essays on Montaigne's representations of aging are those of Bellenger, on the one hand, and Friedrich, on the other. Neither of these works focuses on the cultural implications of Montaigne's representations of aging.
5 In the gerontological literature this is discussed as "dedifferentiation." See Hülür et al.
6 See also Martin et al.
7 See also Thorson and Powell.

Works Cited

Baltes, Paul B. "On the Incomplete Architecture of Human Ontogeny: Selection, Optimization, and Compensation as Foundation of Developmental Theory." *American Psychologist* 52. 4(1997): 366–380.

Bellenger, Yvonne. "Le Thème de la vieillesse dans le livre III des Essais." *Des Signes au sens: Lectures du livre III des Essais. Journées d'Etudes du Centre Montaigne de Bordeaux 14–15 novembre 2002.* Ed. Françoise Argod-Dutard. Paris: Champion, 2003. 201–216.

Cave, Terence. *Thinking with Literature.* Oxford: Oxford UP, 2016.

Cicirelli, Victor G. "Fear of Death in Older Adults: Predictions from Terror Management Theory." *The Journals of Gerontology: Series B* 57. 4(2002): 358–366.

Claus, Karl. "Montaigne on His Essays: Toward a Poetics of the Self." *The Iowa Review* 21. 1(1991): 1–23.

Costello, Matthew C. and Emily K. Bloesch. "Are Older Adults Less Embodied? A Review of Age Effects through the Lens of Cognition." *Frontiers of Psychology* 8 (2017): 1–18.

Erikson, Erik H. *Identity and the Life Cycle.* New York: International UP, 1959.

Foglia, Lucia and Robert A. Wilson. "Embodied Cognition." *Wiley Interdisciplinary Review of Cognitive Science* 4(2013): 319–325.

Friedrich, Hugo. *Montaigne.* Trans. D. Eng. Berkeley: U of California P, 1991.

Greyson, Bruce. "Near-Death Experiences in a Psychiatric Outpatient Clinic Population." *Psychiatric Services* 54. 12(2003): 1649–1651.

Hülür, Gizem, N. Ram, S.L. Willis, K.W. Schaie, and D. Gerstorf. "Cognitive Dedifferentiation with Increasing Age and Proximity of Death: Within-Person Evidence from the Seattle Longitudinal Study." *Psychology and Aging* 30(2015): 311–323.

Johnson, Colleen L., and Barbara M. Barer. *Life Beyond 85 Years: The Aura of Survivorship.* New York: Springer, 1997.

Klencklen, Giuliana, Olivier Després, and André Dufour. "What Do We Know about Aging and Spatial Cognition? Reviews and Perspectives." *Ageing Research Reviews* 11 (2012): 123–135.

Kraft, Eduard. "Cognitive Function, Physical Activity, and Aging: Possible Biological Links and Implications for Multimodal Interventions." *Aging, Neuropsychology, and Cognition* 19(2012): 248–263.

Kübler-Ross, E. *On Death and Dying.* New York: Routledge, 1969.

Martin, Peter, N. Kelly, B. Kahana, E. Kahana, B.J. Willcox, D.C. Willcox, and L.W. Poon. "Definitions of Successful Aging: A Tangible or Elusive Concept?" *The Gerontologist* 55(2015): 14–25.

Mauro, James. "Bright Lights, Big Mystery." *Psychology Today* 25. (July1992): 54–57.

Montaigne, Michel de. *The Complete Essays of Montaigne.* Trans. Donald Frame. Stanford, CA: Stanford UP, 1958.

O'Neill, John. *Essaying Montaigne: A Study of the Renaissance Institution of Writing and Reading.* London: Routledge, 1982.

O'Sullivan, Luke. "'Double et Divers': Writing Doubly in Montaigne's Essais." *The Modern Language Review* 112. 2(2017): 320–340.

Peterson, Nora M. and Peter Martin. "Tracing the Origins of Success: Implications for Successful Aging." *The Gerontologist* 55. 1(2015): 5–13.

Rowe, John W. and Robert L. Kahn. "Successful Aging." *The Gerontologist* 37(1997): 433–440.

Salthouse, Timothy A. "The Processing-Speed Theory of Adult Age Differences in Cognition." *Psychological Review* 103(1996): 403–428.

Skenazi, Cynthia. "The Art of Aging Gracefully: Castiglione's Book of the Courtier and Montaigne's 'On Some Verses of Virgil' (Essays, III, 5)." *Bibliothèque d'Humanisme et Renaissance* 70. 3(2008): 579–593.

Starobinski, Jean. "Montaigne en Mouvement." *Nouvelle Revue française* 15(1960): 16–22.

Staudinger, Ursula M. and Judith Glück. "Psychological Wisdom Research: Commonalities and Differences in a Growing Field." *Annual Review of Psychology* 62(2011): 215–241.

Srivastava, Sanjay, O.P. John, S.D. Gosling, and J. Potter. "Development of Personality in Early and Middle Adulthood: Set Like Plaster or Persistent Change?" *Journal of Personality and Social Psychology* 84. 5(2003): 1041–1053.

Thane, Pat, ed. *The Long History of Old Age.* London: Thames and Hudson, 2005.

Thorson, James A. and F.C. Powell. "Death Anxiety in Younger and Older Adults." *Death Attitudes and the Older Adult: Theories, Concepts, and Applications.* Ed. A. Tomer. Philadelphia: Taylor and Francis, 2000. 123–136.

Tinetti, Mary E. "Performance-Oriented Assessment of Mobility Problems in Elderly Patients." *Journal of the American Geriatric Society* 34(1986): 119–126.

Tornstam, Lars. *Gerotranscendence: A Developmental Theory of Positive Aging.* New York: Springer, 2005.

Yandell, Cathy. "'Corps' and 'Corpus': Montaigne's 'Sur des vers de Virgile'." *Modern Language Studies* 16. 3(1986): 77–87.

Zacks, Rose T. "Working Memory, Comprehension, and Aging: A Review and a New View." *Psychology of Learning and Motivation* 22(1989): 193–225.

12 Witnessing Illness

Phenomenology of Photographic Self Portraiture

Elizabeth Lanphier

Introduction

Photographic self-portraiture as illness narrative situates artist and viewer in an ethical relationship of mutual meaning-making in which other *and* self witness an individual illness experience, and possibly even death. The American performative photographer Hannah Wilke (1940–1993) took such a series of self-portraits during her treatment for terminal lymphoma. Wilke's oeuvre engages with and enacts feminist and phenomenological philosophical concepts. In this respect, her final work, *Intra Venus* is both illness narrative and a fitting culmination of her artistic output.[1] By mobilizing the same themes in *Intra Venus* that preoccupied her larger body of work, Wilke communicates unique, and in some ways provocative, messages about illness. A phenomenological analysis of photography offers insights into the nature of the relationship between a photograph's viewer and the photograph on display. Visual encounters afford a particular kind of knowledge that is both made available and circumscribed by the perspectival limits posed by sight. Photographic self-portraiture is an opportunity for seeing the self as other and sharing a perspective with others. For these reasons the photographic medium offers a unique contribution to a contemporary ethics of care. In an era in which self-portraiture is easily accessible to a general public and woven into social media interactions, these "selfie" images could provide a tool for nurturing ourselves and others, broadening our understanding and experiences of illness, death, and dying.

Hannah Wilke's Art, Philosophy, and Illness

Wilke used her body as a malleable artistic form. Artistically active from the 1960s until her death in 1993, she described her work as "performalist photography" and continually invoked certain personas such as "the angel, the androgyne, the virgin, the goddess, the star" and themes: "gesture, humor, myth, sexuality, narcissism, objecthood, ironic ambiguity and eroticism" (Kochheiser 11). Wilke infused her work with the erotic, melding mind and body, the traditional binary opposition of Cartesian dualism. According to art scholar and Wilke curator, Thomas Kochheiser, Wilke invoked erotic desire as a response to "a capitalistic, totalitarian, religious invention used to control the masses through the denial of the importance of a body language" (141). Erotic desire is central, which speaks to a larger impulse to recognize the role of a body language, or what Maurice Merleau-Ponty might call a body consciousness. When body language or consciousness is foreclosed then the mind achieves a form of totalization, denying the body and taking over as the primary mode of an individual's identity and expression. The erotic refuses this bodily denial and totalization of the mind. Wilke's work, thus, evokes and refutes Cartesian dualism. As she herself notes, "People want others to be the objects of their desire. But I became the subject and the object, objecting to this manipulation" (13).

In *S.O.S. Starification Object Series* (1974), Wilke models her own poses against fashion or women's magazines, evoking several of the personas and themes Kochheiser identifies including the star, objecthood, narcissism, sexuality, and ironic ambiguity. Wilke appears topless, molded into high fashion poses and styles. Wilke herself was quite beautiful, according to mainstream standards. A white woman with long straight hair, high cheekbones, slender figure, hourglass shape, and ample breasts, her beauty rendered her a believable magazine model. However, in each image in *S.O.S. Starification Object Series*, Wilke blemished her body with small folded pieces of chewing gum affixed to her body. These chewing gum "scars" are a version of Wilke's single-folded sculptures, a motif that runs throughout her oeuvre and recalls the look and shape of a clitoris. In this series, they adorn her otherwise perfect skin: one is centered on her forehead, two appear on each cheekbone, and three are evenly spaced across the protruding portion of her chin. The title of the series "Starification" plays on the notions of becoming both a star, and scarred. In the high fashion poses Wilke, performing the role of "star," becomes like the model or movie actress promoting her fame in a glossy magazine.

Yet the blemishes are a type of "scarification," scarring an otherwise idealized image. Thus, Wilke uses visual representation to manifest the physical and psychological malleability expected of women to conform to a culturally dictated ideal and gaze. These photographs of Wilke as glamorous cover girl adorned with single-fold gestural objects, critique female objectification, offering a complicated feminist message about constructions of beauty. Later, Wilke addressed a claim of "narcissism" for featuring her own attractive body in her work:

> People often gave me this bullshit of, "What would you have done if you weren't so gorgeous?" What difference does it make? ... Gorgeous people die as do the stereotypical "ugly." Everybody dies.
>
> (13)

Thus, Wilke's work consciously erodes a strict binary opposition between a tradition where the female form is available for the viewer's gaze and feminism. Wilke controls the gaze that is trained on her. Wilke is not a female object being captured by a male gaze or male artist. Instead she elects what she exposes of herself and directs how she wishes to be seen. Wilke's viewer encounters both her traditional beauty and elements of womanhood, particularly those elements of female pleasure that are normally kept hidden with the overt placement of the single-fold gestural objects. In doing so, Wilke plays with female objectification by drawing the viewer's eye to the clitoris-like images. Instead of being hidden by clothes, pubic hair, or labia, the clitoris is foregrounded by means of sculptural replicas. Wilke takes what is usually interior and hidden and renders it exterior and visible, turning the inside out.

Wilke also collapses oppositional concepts into one another. Her single-fold gestural objects themselves fold in and turn around a single piece of material, literally collapsing outer and inner. The single-fold gestural objects and the conceptual work of *S.O.S. Starification Object Series* each recall Elizabeth Grosz's metaphor of the "Möbius strip" as a way to think about gender as one multisided, continuous thread that turns, twists and folds in on itself.[2] The single-fold gestural objects are a recurring theme in Wilke's work and imagery, appearing within pieces but also as stand-alone sculptures in ceramic, bronze, and latex. These works all invoke fluidity, of concepts, certainly, but also the motion of fluids.

In "Gestures" from 1976, Wilke captures still images of her face in various expressions, images that originated in a 1974 video performance piece. In one piece from "Gestures" there are twelve stills of Wilke arranged in three by four rows, each image related in time to the others yet standing alone, unique among the set. Again there is a complicated fluidity to the images: they are time slices from what would otherwise be a continuous set of movements. On film they would appear entirely fluid, but when frozen in time and extracted in individual photographs they are both continuous and not, related yet separate, individual but a part of a fluid whole.

During 1978–1982 Wilke developed a series of photographs related to her mother, Selma Butter's experience with cancer, including "Portrait of the Artist with her Mother, Selma Butter." The piece includes a topless photograph of Wilke on the left: beautiful, breasts exposed, and purposefully adorned with objects. On the right is a photograph of her mother: also topless, chest exposed, displaying one breast, the other removed from a partial mastectomy. The diptych is both halting and natural. It strikes the viewer with how different the women appear, while fluidly moving between them and their similarities: mother and daughter, young and old, related and separated. Though not known at the time, "Portrait of the Artist with her Mother, Selma Butter," also makes a fluid foreshadowed connection to Wilke's cancer a decade later.

The inversion of interior and exterior as well as the conceptual fluidity of the Möbius strip are replicated in *Intra Venus*, where Wilke takes the private and interior elements of illness and exposes them. We see in *Intra Venus* a prominent place not only for conceptual fluidity, but also for the visual depiction of bodily fluids themselves. Wilke created what turned out to be her final piece (staged posthumously in 1994), over the two years during which she was treated for, and ultimately died from, lymphoma. *Intra Venus* invokes the themes of goddess, myth, sexuality, gesture, narcissism, and objecthood that Wilke deployed throughout her career, now in the context of her own illness. By engaging these personas and themes in this context, Wilke subverts conceptions of illness that exclude beauty, the erotic, or feminine power. She offers a vision of femininity not merely as a vulnerable figure, but as an empowered figure, even during illness.

The photographs that comprise *Intra Venus* display her sick body: naked, ill, sleeping, bathing, on the toilet, in classical poses, in juxtaposition with herself at other moments in time. She shows the body in its decay and demise. And because her work is in dialogue with her body, and her body of work, the images of her infirm body automatically invoke the younger, lithe, healthy body portrayed earlier in her artistic career. Wilke offers her viewer a narrative that includes the path from health to illness, from physical fortitude to physical decline and dependency.

In one self portrait, "Intra-Venus Series #6" Wilke appears in a close up, topless though we see only from her shoulders to the top of her head. She faces the camera, though her head is turned slightly to her right, the viewer's left. She appears to be soaked with water, and her hair hangs straight down, and looks as though it has been brushed down in front of her face. Two things are particularly striking about this image. One is that her hair is quite thin. Though strands remain quite long in front of her face, much of her scalp is visible. Her hair is in the process of thinning and will eventually be lost due to the cancer treatment. The second thing is that the pose recalls her topless glamour headshots in *S.O.S. Starification*. It connects us to Wilke's recent past, her healthy self. In this image from *Intra Venus*, Wilke is also topless, and the pose and cropping of the portrait is similar to what would appear on the cover of a fashion magazine. But here we see that her face is rounder, her body fuller, bloated from fluids or heavier from steroids, in addition to more routine ageing-related weight gain. Instead of the fashion-model smiles that Wilke flashed in *S.O.S. Starification*, here her mouth is downturned, her gaze harder, yet still resolute. Wilke was relatively young (only in her early 50s) when she became ill, so *Intra Venus* represents not a space of time but a gap between health and illness. It reinforces the fluidity between states of health and illness, which might not be separated by much in terms of time or age. This small jump from health to sickness might lead a viewer to reflect on her own embodied self, while reflecting on Wilke.

Wilke molds her sick body into the images of artistic archetypes, deploying poses and imagery that recall the Virgin Mary, the Odalisque, and Ingres paintings (Wilke 11), such as "Intra-Venus (triptych)" which features Wilke naked on a bed of white sheets, adorned only with gauze bandages on her hips and buttocks, and posing like a classical nude painting model. "Intra-Venus Series #1" from July 1992 is a diptych of a self portrait in which Wilke faces the camera straight on. On the left Wilke is seated in what appears like a hospital bed, with a plastic surgical cap on her head, and her shirt open revealing one breast and the ports and tubes that administer her chemotherapy. On the right side is an image of Wilke standing completely naked in a pose that features her voluptuous figure like the *Birth of Venus*. There are wound dressings on both hips, which seem to bookend her curves and genitals more than reflect illness, and she is balancing a flower pot on her head.

These representations are themselves fluid, and the many images depict the body producing fluids and relying on them. "Intra-Venus #1," like many other pictures, shows gauze bandages containing otherwise open wounds, with tubes to ports for IV fluids and chemotherapy. "Intra-Venus #13" contains six separate photographs, two of which include tubes or ports, three of which include bandages, and two that appear to show Wilke on a commode. These photographs do not succumb to shame or embarrassment or to the fluidity of the body: even when vulnerable, Wilke appears not without pride. By embracing and recreating classical artistic references, her photographs illustrate fortitude. The images are beautiful although they defy traditional conceptions of beauty and tackle subjects that are usually kept hidden, or induce shame.

Wilke merges apparent (or potential) opposites, complicates them, and does not allow for them to be (dualistically) either subverted or contained. Wilke already provoked the cohabitation of opposing ideas in her work challenging beauty standards and female objectification. Just as she refuted idealized notions of female beauty in her "Starification Series" and other works, this subtle subversion was nonetheless conducted on the site of her attractive body and image. Wilke played upon female objectification, deployed it, and in this manner contained the trope of woman-as-object-to-be-viewed. Yet by upending the expectations attendant on a beautiful female image she also subverted these hypocritical standards. Similarly, with her illness experience, she makes a space in which the beautiful and the ugly, the vulnerable and the proud, are held together and are in fact more starkly revealed due to the co-existence of their opposite. Wilke tells a more complicated illness narrative than the three types that Arthur Frank has enumerated: quest, chaos, or restitution narrative. Wilke's work displays elements of all three narrative types as she tries to make sense of the chaotic experience of illness and reclaim agency over her life, yet she transcends them by portraying herself as a goddess, the Virgin Mary, and a mythical woman with superhuman stories.

The very title *Intra Venus* comingles ideas and meaning, a pun on "intravenous," alluding to a medical narrative, while invoking the myth, love, beauty, and sexuality associated with the goddess Venus. This mythical allusion situates *Intra Venus* in the art historical pantheon, with the *Venus de Milo* and Botticelli's *The Birth of Venus*. Yet being "intra" Venus reveals another Möbius strip of interior and exterior folding in on each other. Is Venus inside Wilke? Is Wilke inside Venus? Is it the beauty within or is she within beauty? The dichotomies of interior/exterior, ugly/beautiful, sick/healthy, are rendered complex, fluid, confused. *Intra Venus* philosophically responds to and refutes a Cartesian, dualistic separation of mind/body, health/illness, self/other. Thereby, Wilke gives her audience the opportunity to confront suffering through a visual, understandable illness narrative. Everyone's body dies, but Wilke calls upon her audience to bear witness not to an abstract "death" but to individual suffering. Her art enacts a poignant philosophy of particularity and an imperative for an ethics of relationality, and perhaps even care.

Phenomenology, Photography, Self, and Other

Wilke's artwork demands a hermeneutical engagement, requiring its participants (maker and viewer) to engage in philosophical reflection. In this regard Wilke's art engages philosophically, rather than being an illustrative instantiation of philosophical concepts. In other words, Wilke's art can be said to deepen philosophical thinking rather than merely depict it. If she saw herself as a "performalist" photographer, we might also view her as a "performalist" philosopher, working in both phenomenological and feminist traditions.

Feminist philosophers comment on the need for first-person, situated accounts in philosophy to combat the illusion that all experience, therefore all philosophy, is, or can be, universal. Wilke's art is just such an account, especially of illness as part of a relational ethics or ethics of care. Wilke's art enacts, performs, calls its artist and viewer into an ethical relationship toward each other of mutual meaning-making, awareness of subjectivity, and inter-subjectivity. Furthermore, the achievement of her artistic illness narrative paves the way for additional first-personal photographic illness narratives as tools to deepen an ethics of care, which prioritizes relationships and the traits that follow from interpersonal relationships, such as dependency, vulnerability, responsibility, trust, friendship, love, empathy, and compassion.

None of this is to say that Wilke thought she was presenting an "authentic" self. Art historian Amelia Jones notes that the photographs are "insufficient as replacements for the subject 'Hannah Wilke,'" commenting on "the failure of photography to sustain a relation to the 'authentic' self" (in Wilke 13). Yet Wilke was not attempting to generate the authentic self; her art is phenomenologically coherent because the representation could not stand in for the embodied self. In the *Intra Venus* catalogue, Wilke's husband, Donald Goddard, noted that she intended to write what Arthur Frank might describe as a restitution narrative. Her working title was "Cured," though Goddard acknowledged that Wilke knew, long before she finished *Intra Venus,* that the restitution narrative outlined by the title would not come to fruition (Wilke 16).

Merleau-Ponty says "to look at an object is to inhabit it" (79). Contemporary phenomenologist Alfonso Lingis writes in *The Imperative* that our body image comes not from internal imagination but from our own gazing at others; Lingis echoes and builds upon Merleau-Ponty by suggesting that "to look is to become visible" (62). Lingis conceptually deepens intersubjective perception embodiment: Perception is not only our own awareness of our embodiment or our encounter with the embodiment of others and our awareness of their embodiment; our perception of others also generates our embodied awareness of ourselves. Wilke, in capturing herself as object and making herself the viewing subject, therefore becomes visible. And arguably, if "to look is to become visible," then Wilke renders her viewer visible through the viewer's act of looking at her image. The occasion of viewing Wilke's art, of encountering and *looking* at it, is an occasion for the viewer to perceive her own embodiment. Furthermore, in documenting herself, she gives her audience a concept of their selfhood as audience that they would not otherwise possess in this particular moment: only in relation to a piece of art can the viewer become an audience. Subject and object, the onlooker and the one being looked at, are bridged in the artistic space: both viewer and the one being viewed, while each from their own perspectives, inhabit (in part) the object, or empathize with its experience. Wilke's photographic artwork could be seen to confuse the binary opposition of subject–object.

Wilke's refusal of binary assignations complicates the ways in which we regard the self, the other, and the self as other. And art complicates these dialectical relationships because the piece of art produced is a third type of entity with which other selves engage. The meaning of this third entity is constantly produced and reproduced in each instance of reception. Even for a piece of static visual art deemed "finished" and presented to an audience, each new view or viewer creates an element of seeing anew, creating new meaning, and a unique hermeneutical experience. Arguably, the ongoing work of meaning-making occurs after art is presented to an audience, for only "once images are made public," can "they become freed from the motivations and subjectivity of those responsible for their creation and enter an inter-subjective world where interpretations are open to all" (Richards, Warren, and Gott 69). In other words, the full expression of an artwork is only, and repeatedly, achieved as this third entity co-constructed between artist and viewer. Furthermore, because that said encounter has a temporal component, the meaning of the art is mutable. A piece of art's meaning will be fluid from viewer to viewer, but also potentially from instance of viewing to instance of viewing for the same viewer.

The images in *Intra Venus* are at times difficult to view because they viscerally reveal frank and intimate experiences of illness. Yet despite their challenging subject matter they remain beautiful and engaging. Lingis writes that "to face an other is to touch with the eyes ... the bruises and calluses of the one who has presented ... herself" (131). Lingis suggests a tangibility to the way the other is able to perceive the "suffering of another" which can be "felt in our eyes" not "at a viewing distance" but in "our sensibility immediately" (132). Read through Lingis, *Intra Venus* is Wilke presenting the viewer with a palpable understanding of her suffering, which "afflicts" the viewer's sensibility (Lingis 132) like lymphoma afflicts Wilke's own body. Wilke presents herself to her audience, enabling viewers to "touch with the eyes" her suffering, her "bruises and calluses," her disease.

As Lingis observes, to "face an other" is not only to "touch" and to "feel" but also "to hear" (131) and "to speak is to respond to someone who has presented himself or herself" (135). A question then regarding Wilke is: to whom is she responding? Has Wilke called to her audience to speak for her in her absence, when she has been silenced by death? A viewer cannot stand in for

Wilke; the audience will regard her from their own embodied position. Here we might think of Heidegger and being-toward-death as what makes our *Dasein*: we each must die our particular death. According to Heidegger's account, witnessing the death of another is not instructive regarding our own death, which is always singular. In regarding Wilke's dying process in pictures we are not learning what it is like to die ourselves. We are learning what illness and dying are like *for her*. Yet if "to look at an object is to inhabit it" (Merleau-Ponty 79) then Wilke invites her audience into her home to inhabit being-toward-death with her. Additionally, while Wilke was living, her pictures were objects that she too could look at and inhabit. Thus she was able to share a perspective with her audience, though temporarily. Wilke created a kind of (artistic) encounter that persists beyond her death. She created the possibility for repeated encounters in which the art and its viewer exist (in being-toward-death), and co-construct meaning, together, although she is gone.

Sharing Perspectives: The Phenomenology of Self Portraiture

In directing her viewers' gaze toward her art, Wilke directs their gaze toward her body, not only breaking down dichotomous thinking but also challenging dialectical thinking. Multiple participants engage with the work: Wilke as photographer (the self); the audience viewing her work (the other) in a gallery, museum, or publication; and Wilke the photographer looking at Wilke the photographic subject (self-looking-back-at-the-self). Wilke was part of the audience of her images and could see the self from a shared perspective that she invited others to see. By turning the camera on herself, Wilke is in the unique situation of being able to enact the roles of artist, subject, and viewer. And it is in this realm of the self-looking-back-at-the-self, assuming the gaze of the other, in which totalization, or the absorption of one into another, is impossible. In a Hegelian dialectical system, two opposing forces are in dialogue: one is the thesis, the other is the antithesis, and if their opposition is resolved it is a form of synthesis. However this synthesis has a totalizing effect: the thesis and antithesis are no longer independent; they have been fused together into a (totalizing) synthesis. In Wilke's photographic self-portraits there is the self (thesis), and the other (antithesis). Yet the photograph is not the synthesis, but instead a more permeable, many layered, or many-*leveled* (to use Lingis's phrase) experience. By turning the camera on her own body, Wilke may witness how her body is viewed by the other when being-for-others. In making her body her subject, she is at once for herself and for others.

Merleau-Ponty notes that "the body is to be compared, not to a physical object, but rather to a work of art" and that some ideas are "incommunicable by means other than the display of colors and sounds" (174). So in rendering the self as (photographic) object, the self is made into a work of art, a "representation" to be interpreted by the other. Yet, for Merleau-Ponty this could not be "a representation like any other" in part because the body is not "an object like any other" (109). The body can be represented, but this representation is not an objective means of experience for "I cannot understand the function of the living body except by enacting it myself, and except in so far as I am a body which rises toward the world" (Merleau-Ponty 87). The self understands a body by having one; identity is generated by embodiment, for "we are literally what others think of us and what our world is" (122).

Thus we are for ourselves, but we are also what we are for others, and this way of being-for-others is something we can never quite experience in ourselves. Merleau-Ponty writes, "I am not in front of my body, I am in it, or rather I am it" (173). The self cannot get in front of its own body to regard it with the gaze of the other. Even facing a mirror and seeing back our reflection we see a version of ourselves unlike what others see of us, for the image is reversed. So although the self experiences herself from her own unique embodied position, others also experience us from their own unique embodied position. They see a version of us that we cannot see ourselves.

Artistic representation of the self is not the embodied self, but a second-order experience of the self. Merleau-Ponty describes how looking in a mirror does not allow one to step outside embodied experience, for instance. Yet, while Wilke cannot regard her *embodied* self as another can, her art permits *some* encounter with the experience of how the other regards the self beyond the embodied position. It is not that Wilke creates a representation of herself which she can see (indeed, this representation is an ersatz reproduction), but rather that in creating art for an audience, she creates a new mode of engagement with her body in an artistic space.

The body in a photograph is neither self nor other, it is an entirely new production. Artist and audience gaze upon the work in a particular shared experience of intersecting time and place created by an artistic encounter. Importantly, both the self-body represented, and the audience regarding it, are necessary for art to be recognized and experienced as such: their individual experiences are vulnerable to the other because they rely on the other to constitute them as artist or as audience.

In one respect, Wilke was speaking to herself. In the *Intra Venus* catalogue Amelia Jones discusses Wilke's historical relationship to narcissism. Jones comments that Narcissus "both *wants* himself and *is* himself and yet becomes *not himself* through his own desire" (Wilke 6). Similarly, Wilke represents herself, yet is herself, and becomes something else (the object) to both herself and the other, as something other than herself, the image in the picture. Jones suggests that Wilke employed "photography to objectify her body for herself" as a way to "make the signs of cancer and its treatments legible: to make sense of death" (Wilke 12).

Hannah Wilke can render herself visible as her own subject and object; however, death is an event we cannot render visible to ourselves. Levinas writes, "the death of the other is an *end,* the point at which the separated being is cast in to the totality" and "*dying* can be passed through the past" (56). Heidegger identifies the deaths of other beings as instructive as to what it is like for others to die, but says they do not teach us what it is like for us to die our own deaths. Death remains phenomenologically inaccessible from a first-person standpoint. We cannot experience dying as our *own* endpoint until we die. Thus, Wilke cannot make her *own* death legible even by turning the camera lens on herself. In documenting her disease, she depicts what Levinas calls "coming to an end" (56) but not the moment she will come to an end. Yet, in approaching both herself and her death as photographic objects, she documents a view that approaches, but does not fully achieve, the gaze of the self normally witnessed only by the other. Art gets her closer to witnessing her own demise.

Conclusion: Self, Selfie, and Others

I suggest above that elements of Wilke's art function as a feminist artistic critique that destabilizes traditional gender binaries. I have further suggested that *Intra Venus* deepens Wilke's disruption of binary thinking around illness in addition to gender. *Intra Venus* acts as illness narrative and philosophical product, in which Wilke places disease in dialogue with art, history, and beauty. I claim that art creates an intersubjective hermeneutic in which art(ist) and viewer remain in a dialectical relationship co-constructing a meaning that is unique to a particular encounter in time, place, and viewership. Wilke's deployment of photographic self-portraiture complicates this dialectic by allowing Wilke to regard herself, as her audience does, and bear witness to her own suffering, illness, and being-toward-death.

In an era of "selfie culture," individuals routinely turn their cameras (or smartphones) on themselves and disseminate carefully curated pictures on various social media platforms. Some might lament this apparently narcissistic trend, or critique the ways the "self" in selfies is a highly constructed, incomplete portrait. More optimistically, the methods and lessons of Wilke's work might be used to reflect on how we co-construct meaning with others and ourselves in photographs, and that this opportunity to witness ourselves and others could inform ethical care.

Selfies present an opportunity. They provide a tool for personalizing experiences and confronting ourselves and others with images that draw us into ethical relations of mutual meaning-making, care, and understanding. Yet they also pose a risk. For the lesson we learn from Wilke is that this kind of project requires a radical vulnerability. Wilke carefully crafted her image in these photographs. Yet while they invoke the beauty of Venus and the history of art, she also chose to display her body in scenes of intense vulnerability: sick, naked, bloated, fluid. The ethical work of selfies as co-constructed narrative requires a willingness to be vulnerable, and to offer vulnerable images of oneself to both others and the self. Taking images of what would normally only remain interior, the private and vulnerable moments, and making them exterior through self-portraiture, enters them into an intersubjective space for interpretation, identification, imagination, and affiliation.

Although the kind of self-portraiture Wilke presented in *Intra Venus* could invite criticism, or might cause its viewer to turn away at times in shame or disgust, her artistry captivates her audience, guiding her viewer's gaze back to the work. And this gaze opens up an opportunity for attention and presence, in which the viewer is present with Wilke in her illness experience. It is through her vulnerability that Wilke creates a possibility for both understanding, and care, between herself and her viewer. Photographic self-portraiture as illness narrative offers a powerful tool for understanding the self, the other, and the illness experience. The making, witnessing, and reception of *Intra Venus* enact a practice of narrative medicine, engaging its core principles of attention, representation, and affiliation that Rita Charon has identified as part of telling and receiving stories of illness both inside and outside of medical institutions. Wilke trains her own gaze and that of her audience on her illness, commanding attention. She represents herself and her illness through both beautiful and vulnerable imagery. And she invites her audience to affiliate with her, to recognize her illness experience as both particular to her and universal to the process of living and dying. *Intra Venus* illustrates the power of illness narratives and the unique possibilities of photography as a narrative device.

Notes

1 Except for Tamar Tembeck's analysis of Wilke's work as "photographic autopathography," most other scholarship discusses her work as part of a radical feminist American art movement rather than as an illness narrative.
2 Gender is a complex and actively theorized concept. My aim here is merely to suggest that Wilke's work can be read as a feminist critique of dualism.

Works Cited

Charon, Rita. *Narrative Medicine: Honoring the Stories of Illness*. New York: Oxford UP, 2008.
Frank, Arthur. *The Wounded Storyteller: Body, Illness and Ethics*. Chicago, IL: U of Chicago P, 1995.
Grosz, Elizabeth. *Volatile Bodies*. Bloomington: Indiana UP, 1994.
Hegel, Georg Wilhelm Friedrich. *Phenomenology of Spirit*. Trans. A.V. Miller. Oxford: Oxford UP, 1977.
Heidegger, Martin. *Being and Time*. Trans. John Macquarrie and Edward Robinson. New York: Harper Perennial, 2008.
Kochheiser, Thomas, ed. *Hannah Wilke: A Retrospective*. Columbia: U of Missouri P, 1989.
Levinas, Emmanuel. *Totality and Infinity*. Trans. Alphonso Lingis. Pittsburgh: Duquesne UP, 1961.
Lingis, Alphonso. *The Imperative*. Bloomington: Indiana UP, 1998.
Merleau-Ponty, Maurice. *Phenomenology of Perception*. Trans. Colin Smith. New York: Routledge Classics, 2002.
Richards, Naomi, Lorna Warren, and Merryn Gott. "The Challenge of Creating 'Alternative' Images of Ageing: Lessons from a Project with Older Women." *Journal of Aging Studies* 26(2012): 65–78.
Tembeck, Tamark. "Exposed Wounds: The Photographic Autopathographies of Hannah Wilke and Jo Spence." *Canadian Art Review* 33. 1/2(2003): 87–101.
Wilke, Hannah. *Intra Venus*. New York: Ronald Feldmen Fine Arts, 1995.

13 Disjunction and Relationality in Terminal Illness Writing

Yianna Liatsos

In August 2008, after being rushed to the emergency room with a seizure, British art critic Tom Lubbock was diagnosed with terminal Glioblastoma Multiforme (GBM), the most aggressive primary malignancy of the central nervous system. In the wake of this diagnosis, Lubbock and his wife, artist Marion Coutts, each wrote a memoir about their experience: Lubbock's *Until Further Notice I am Alive* was published in 2012 and Coutts' *The Iceberg* appeared in 2014. These two texts constitute a remarkable literary event not only because of their quality (each garnered critical accolades and Coutts' book won the 2015 Wellcome Prize), but also because their combination affords us a unique opportunity to explore the greater narrative ecology of illness. If illness writing, as Neil Vickers has noted in his recent review of the genre, incorporates narratives composed both by patients and caregivers, then Lubbock's and Coutts' memoirs illuminate the singularity of each of these two subject positions in illness writing, as well as their entanglement. Through their respective books on the experience of the same terminal cancer diagnosis, these two "wounded storytellers," to use Arthur Frank's phrase, point to the temporal correspondences and disjunctions and the interrelational affinities and disconnect of their shared life with illness.[1]

The temporal horizon and relational textuality of these two memoirs invites a critical constellation of two philosophical concepts that have substantial bearing on a discussion of illness narrative, those of "transformative experience" (L.A. Paul and Havi Carel) and of the "interrelational dimension of selfhood" (Adriana Cavarero and Judith Butler). Carel has grappled with the radical changes that illness inaugurates and has employed Paul's notion of "transformative experience" to address how epistemologically and existentially life-changing the experience of serious illness can be for the patient—so much so, according to Carel, that neither primary caregivers nor readers of illness narratives can access the experience of illness as such. Butler, on the other hand, has turned to Cavarero's discussion of the interpersonal dimension of selfhood, to consider the individual self as inherently dependent on and realizable through others, while being opaque to itself. Lubbock's and Coutts' memoirs expand on these contending philosophical positions by bringing the full weight of an aggressive terminal diagnosis to bear on the patient's and on the primary caregiver's narrative identities. These two illness narratives, in their respective experience of the embodied self in time and its corresponding relation to language, also engage with and complicate the opacity at the heart of self-referential writing and relational ethics.

"Cancer scarcely allows you time to look at it, let alone get used to it," says Coutts in her memoir (122). S. Lochlann Jain has written about the temporal experience of cancer by naming it "living in prognosis" and noting how the prognostic charts associated with one's cancer diagnosis sever the experience of the normative, developmental timeline, even as they offer new versions of time to live in.[2] The effects of this new temporality in the context of a particularly catastrophic prognosis, to use Coutts' term for GBM, become a central preoccupation in both Lubbock's and Coutts' memoirs. Dubbed by neurosurgeon Eric Holland "the terminator," GBM has a *median* survival of 3 months if untreated and 14.6 months among patients who follow the standard treatments for "managing" the tumor through radical tumor resection, chemotherapy, and radiotherapy (Lacroix et al.). The fast pace of GBM's growth, in addition to the significant morbidity associated with its progression (that entails increasingly worsening symptoms of neurological, cognitive, and other physical decline), complicates treatment and care for the same reason that it troubles the registration of illness-as-experience in a meaning-inducing way (Lacroix et al.). If, as Hayden White has asserted, narrative emplotment endows human experience with meaning unlike annals or chronicles that only list events, it also necessitates the kind of critical distance afforded by time (6). In the context of what Coutts describes as "a high-speed disease with full, motorway pile-up repercussions," the possibility of narrativity becomes tenuous at best, and in the case of Lubbock's and Coutts' memoirs writing takes on an episodic quality that lacks the editorial prowess of hindsight, or the culminating promise of clarity and actualization (122). Put simply, the truncated temporality that GBM and other aggressive illnesses beget curtails introspection's potential for clarifying reality and meaning, a predicament that has added repercussions when it comes to end-of-life considerations.[3] Instead, this temporality of perpetual shock generates a kind of opacity that in Lubbock's memoir is associated with the materiality of a disintegrating body, while in Coutts' text is linked to the task of being a primary witness to what she describes as "the obliteration of a person, his intellect, his experience, his agency" (90).

Lubbock's *Until Further Notice I am Alive* consists of diary entries that date from "August 2008" to "October 2010," that is from the month when an unprecedented "fit" first brought him to an emergency room for observation and tests until the month when his decline "signaled the end of home," as Coutts writes in her introduction to her husband's slim memoir.[4] Both the style and the title of Lubbock's book convey his relationship to his writing, which is as open-ended as it is jarringly present. The memoir's first two lines communicate an unequivocal sense of his diagnosis' prognostic implications: "The news was death," Lubbock writes. "And it wasn't going to be maybe good luck and getting through it. It was definitely death, and quite soon" (11). What ensues is writing that endeavors to work through this definitive lack of future, which as Lubbock himself notes and as literary scholar and memoirist Nancy

K. Miller has suggested, undoes the very foundation that makes narrative possible.[5] In Lubbock's memoir the repetition of particular concerns, oftentimes producing contradictory conclusions, indicates an unsteady narrative short-term memory that can be read as a textual effect of the foreclosed future. "One blessing at the moment," Lubbock says early in his memoir, before the first of his two brain surgeries, is "being let off from having to think about the future, from making plans, projects" (18). Relieved of what he calls "futuremindedness," Lubbock observes himself as being "in a more productive state of mind" (18). When he receives the definitive GBM prognosis following the craniotomy however ("the results are ... as bad as they can be. The most active level of malignancy. Very quick-growing"), Lubbock predicts the impossibility of preparing himself for death, precisely because futuremindedness is un-relievable (36): "when the forking of paths approaches, I will find that I cannot remotely imagine it, and can only imagine a future of life," he concedes (38). In the same diary entry (dated 8 October 2008) he consoles himself by considering "the human *practice* of dying" and resolving that the course one should follow is to "hold your allegiance to the world, even while accepting your links to it are very weak" (40). A fortnight later (entry dated 19 October 2008) he grieves losing "the indefinite, open-ended prospect of life," its "ongoingness" as he calls it. Without it, he notes, "our life appears alien" (47).

The alienation Lubbock points to here returns to the foundational philosophical schism between mind and body, between consciousness driven to establish sense and meaning through order and control, while the "body in all its ways ... prosaic, material, solid, opaque, secular, untranscendent, this-worldly" governs existence according to its own anarchic carnality (20).[6] In one of the early entries Lubbock describes the task of accommodating this split, and the "alien life" it can produce, as a lesson he tries to teach himself, "a lesson in imagination, in self-imagination" (46). Described in this way, and coupled with Coutts' description of death as being personal ("Tom was no exception," she notes), Lubbock's memoir can be read as an attempt to work through what Carel, via Paul, has described as the transformational radicality of illness—its ultimate manifestation, according to Paul, being the experience of death (7).[7] Paul's book, entitled *Transformative Experience* (2014), is preoccupied with normative decision theory. Paul considers the kind of lived experience that dramatically reorients one to life and to oneself in an effort to expose the limits of a rational choice, with its dependence on predictable outcomes. First describing an "epistemically" transformative experience as the kind that changes one's subjective view,[8] Paul proceeds to discuss the "personally" transformative experience as:

> life-changing in [a way] that changes what it is like for you to be you, that is, it can change your point of view ... your personal preferences, and perhaps even change the kind of person that you are or at least take yourself to be.
>
> (16)

Carel employs Paul's concept to address the personally transformative quality of illness and insists on its epistemic inaccessibility to those who have not undergone this experience or received a diagnosis of serious—terminal—illness. "To deeply care for and mourn an ill person's losses and suffering," Carel notes:

> can teach us much about illness. Moreover, reading accounts of illness can both edify and inform non-patients about the experience of illness. ... But to know, fully and first-hand, what it is like to have a serious illness, to experience bodily failure, vulnerability, and anxiety about one's body and one's life, one needs to have the experience itself.
>
> (Carel, Kidd, and Pettigrew 1152)

Lubbock's perspective on his illness as a lesson in *self*-imagination, then, echoes Carel's insight into the singularity of the experience for the patient.

Illness memoirs are replete with claims that hint at such radical departure of lived experience and personal identity, even as they proceed to trace the contours of the experience for their readers. Individually, this understanding of illness's experiential inaccessibility posits the predicament of how the self, in confrontation with such radical newness, can begin to register and comprehend itself: from what position does the "new" self begin to register the newness of the experience if not from the position of, or in collaboration with the "old" self? Collectively, this understanding posits the predicament or relationality and communication within the larger domain of illness—an issue that is at the heart of medical and health humanities and is the foundation of the pedagogical discourse of narrative medicine. How can an experience that can only be known by the patient be meaningfully communicated to medical staff and to caregivers who do not have the experience? What might it mean to try and ameliorate patient care in the context of this impasse?

Cavarero's insight into the fundamental interrelationality of selfhood appears to provide a much-needed balance to the absoluteness of illness's singularity, offering a perspective that illuminates the relationship between a terminally ill patient and, in the context of this chapter, his primary caregiver and advocate. Selfhood, for Cavarero, is founded on the exposure—visibility—of corporeality that makes it both inherently singular (precisely because the embodied exposure renders it irreducible) and dependent (precisely because the exposure necessitates an other who will recognize it). For Cavarero, an ethics of relation that emerges from this perspective of selfhood "does not support empathy, identification, or confusion," but instead recognizes "the necessary other as a finitude that remains irremediably an other in all the fragile and unjudgeable insubstitutability of her existing" (92). In addressing the self through this exchange, which she links to the telling of one's story, Cavarero offers a poignant insight for understanding the shared narrative scene that Lubbock's and Coutts' memoirs forge. Without relinquishing the uniqueness of either author, Cavarero allows their reciprocal exposition as distinct selves, whereby Lubbock's story is never reduced to Coutts' story (and vice versa), but neither do the two selves become solipsistic. Butler takes Cavarero's insight further. If the self depends on its exposure to the other for a sense of itself (via the process of recognition that unfolds in the scene of address), then it is also fundamentally vulnerable to the other and opaque to itself. The self's exteriority produces an opacity of the conditions of its emergence and thus of a central dimension of the self's singularity. "If it is precisely by virtue of one's relations to others that one is opaque to oneself," Butler argues, "and if those relations to others are the venue of one's ethical responsibility, then it may well follow that it is precisely by virtue of the subject's opacity to itself that it incurs and sustains some of its most important ethical bonds" (20). This insight into the fundamental opacity of the self for-itself becomes decidedly relevant in the case of a patient who is given a fast-paced terminal diagnosis that entails the gradual loss of his cognitive abilities, even as it is further complicated by the ethical demands that such opacity raises for the greater illness community. If one of the most devastating effects of GBM's progression entails precisely this thickening of impenetrability that Butler describes as "the subject's opacity to itself," what might it mean for the subject's medical and intimate caregivers, and for the readers of his memoir, to attend to this opacity as it begins to consume the subject? To paraphrase Ludwig Wittgenstein's question raised by Lubbock in the final diary entry of his memoir, what might it mean to care for a patient who can no longer speak an audible language but who may still say things to himself in his—inaudible, opaque—imagination? Lubbock's and Coutts' memoirs engage these quandaries by describing their respective transformative experience as giving rise to a multifaceted consciousness with distinct parameters regarding the self and the world, some parts of which become relatable and communicable while others remain opaque and aphasic.

We have already seen how the new temporality that the diagnosis of GBM inaugurates produces a vacillating perspective. *Until Further Notice* embodies this struggle, lyrically encapsulated in Lubbock's claim that the "shape of the creature is the pressure of life against the limit of death" (53). The book's shifting textuality reveals the prognostic effects in its author's thinking, which is also affected by physiological changes and pharmaceutical side effects that Lubbock is living through and frequently considers. "Teaching dying," he notes, "if it could be done, would be in part to teach you how to keep your view on both life and death" (50). Lubbock's memoir, with its efforts at self-imagination in the face of dying, becomes a manual of double-consciousness that doggedly contains the two warring trajectories of prospect and availability. Through his writing this consciousness assumes both ordinary and apocalyptic forms, upholding hope while remaining autothanatographical.[9] Early in his diagnosis Lubbock adopts a composed perspective to express satiability with what life has offered in terms of love and work, noting that in respect to the bad news he has received, "extinction in itself is not [his] grief" (38). Two weeks later, while in the throes of the agonizing realization of an encroaching death, he considers the merit of suicide: "Suppose I said: I can't stand it," he reflects, "what would I do? ... There are no terms to ... come to. I could kill myself, so as to escape the intolerability of dying" (49). Similarly, the letters he writes to his wife and son before his first brain surgery (dated 29 September 2008) assume the detached and thoughtful tone of a sendoff informed by a resolute surrender to the possibility of death: "How sure I am that you and he, together and in your individual selves, will go on well. ... What a fantastic pleasure it's been so far," he writes to Coutts (27). The epistolary diary entry he writes to his wife before the second brain surgery however (dated 12 April 2010) expresses far more frailty and supplication: "all I want is: prolong, prolong—though of course an open-ended life would suit us so much better" (107).[10]

The doubleness that is traceable in Lubbock's memoir then entails, on the one hand, a kind of surrender to the disease's foreclosed futurity and collapsing carnal vectors that entail a deepening opacity; and on the other hand attentiveness to the physical and emotional attachment he has with Coutts and their son, that is, the interrelational dimension of selfhood's intimate exposure. In fact the very title of his book is inspired by Coutt's obstinate invitation at future relationality in the face of Lubbock's GBM diagnosis, shared in an anecdote he tells his friends in one of the regular emails he sends them to keep them informed of his condition (this one dated 20 October 2008):

> this evening Marion said to me: you do know that I fully intend to be with you for another ten years (she had seen how my thoughts were tending) and I could only answer: yes, why the hell not! Of course, I can't help considering all my worst possibilities, but I've probably too quickly adopted the role of moribund. So until further notice, I am alive.
>
> (48)

Coutts' own experience of being her husband's primary caregiver during the thirty months he lives with GBM is movingly and incompletely captured here by Lubbock. In Lubbock's memoir Coutts appears as the warrior partner who replies "OK I'm on it" upon receiving the news of Lubbock's brain tumour, even if she first gasps and weeps (13). "Marion holds us all together," he writes in his final email to his friends (dated 1 September 2010) (Coutts 186). Coutts herself confirms adopting this role in her own memoir: "I am an over-achiever," she declares midway through *The Iceberg*, at the same time that Lubbock's memoir concludes (in August 2010, when he ends his diary entries): "I will do anything and everything and all," she adds (126). One does not have to look very far before or after this declaration, however, to find writing that expresses uncertainty and precariousness in the face of Lubbock's pending loss.

Coutts' memoir traverses the same time span and space as Lubbock's but is made up of numbered sections and subsections that signal a kind of narrative ordering, however minimal, conferred by retrospection, even as the book opens with the oracular assertion "A book about the future must be written in advance. Later I won't have the energy to speak. So I will do it now" (1). In her "5x15" talk of *The Iceberg* Coutts noted how her original writing began at a "violent" and "volatile" time during Lubbock's illness, and emulated the violent character of its context by assuming the form of scattered textual fragments that functioned as "a reflex action, like spitting or pointing or trying to grab at something."[11] In her effort to turn these pieces into a book she edited and expanded them, while guarding the fierce physicality of the original bricolage and choosing fidelity to the temporality of her experience, which echoed the unremitting linear march from Lubbock's diagnosis until his death. The published book captures the simultaneous editorial authority and the immediacy of the present continuous that shapes the reality of the caregiver whose loved one declines before her eyes. If serious illness begets a transformative experience that is the patient's alone, as Carel suggests, then Coutts' memoir reveals how it also begets a transformative experience that is the primary caregiver's alone.

Coutts encapsulates the clash between these temporalities as "the steadiness of the quotidian and the crash-consciousness of its ending" (49). In exploring the effects of what in medical parlance has been dubbed "anticipatory grief," Coutts' *The Iceberg* complicates even as it upholds the affirmation of presence that *Until Further Notice I Am Alive* articulates. In addressing the experience of the caregiver Coutts' memoir depicts how readily she assumes the responsibilities of caring for Lubbock, while nonetheless remaining inherently blind to what lies ahead, positioned as she is "at the heart of the gathering chaos" (50). Being a caregiver, Coutts says, entails knowing that you are nearing an iceberg whose full depth and scope and potential for damage you can never know in advance of crashing into it, elucidating here Carel's insight about the quality of illness's transformative experience by identifying its concealed ferocity. Where Lubbock's memoir captures the uncanny experience of terminal illness's initiation of a double consciousness associated with living and dying, Coutts' memoir describes a different type of double consciousness—indeed more a triple, even quadruple consciousness—which has to do with simultaneously maintaining vigilance over the patient's "prognostic" temporality of cancer, while anticipating the possible futures and preparing for different eventualities. Where Lubbock "has the sword and mighty shield, the gravitas of the seriously ill," Coutts notes, her own job as the commentator, as "the wholly partial observer," is a position that is unarmed and thus "further out in danger"— something that Coutts claims both she and Lubbock acknowledge (49).

The elucidation of this cryptic claim can be found in almost every page of Coutts' memoir, and essentially revolves around her work as a caregiver, which she describes as a threefold task:

1 Not to let Tom be destroyed before his death but to help him live it fully in his own way with all his power.
2 Not to let Ev be destroyed by Tom's death but to help him live it fully in his own way with all his power.
3 Not to let myself be destroyed. See 1 and 2.

(125)

Coutts' violent wavering between her attentiveness to her husband's and son's absolute need for care and her own individual opacity ("it is impossible to explain my strategy … it is opaque even to me" she says), gives her reader a sense of what the caregiver's danger entails (73). For Coutts, her nuclear family or "unit," as she calls it, comprised of Lubbock, herself, and their 18 month-old son Ev, is both the ground zero of the GBM catastrophe and the sole ground on which to stand. "The news makes a rupture with what went before," Coutts notes about Lubbock's GBM diagnosis early in her memoir, "clean, complete and total save in one respect. It seems that after the event, the decision we make is to remain. Our unit stands. This alone will not save us but whenever we look, it is the case" (1–2). The role of the unit and its power pertains to the embodied exposure and recognition described by Cavarero. In the in-flux time of illness's rupture, the unit provides the fixed referent that grounds Lubbock and Coutts alike, albeit erratically, since both Lubbock and Ev are in an active process of transforming in opposite directions, one toward disintegration, the other toward individuation (2). The anxiety and solitude Coutts experiences in caring for each of them alone is powerfully captured in her brief reference to financial worries that she begins to develop in relation to Lubbock's treatment and the family's short-term (with Lubbock) and long-term (without Lubbock) future. When after Lubbock's second craniotomy Coutts describes waking up soaked in a sweat of ice from money worries and "feebly starting up conversations" about the matter, she notes how Lubbock "has no interest in these conversations" (109). "His concerns are not these," she admits. "This is so understandable that I abandon my case" (109). The affective impact of this tension is nowhere sharper, however, than in Coutts' impassive description of the tasks at hand during the last autumn of Lubbock's life (he died on 9 January 2011). She writes "my task this month is twofold. I need to find somewhere for my husband to die and I need to find a primary school for my child. The deadline for both is now" (244).

One of the textual differences in Coutts' description of being the primary caregiver to Lubbock versus Ev is that in the case of the former, she often employs the collective pronoun "we" to qualify their shared experience. Cavarero has discussed the use of the collective "we" pronoun in the context of relational narrative ethics as an ontological error, and Carel has addressed it as an epistemological one in the context of the illness experience. Coutts' memoir very deliberately employs the collective "we" to express what appears to be a visceral solidarity. This "we" is formulated from the first page of Coutt's memoir, where she uses a kind of syncopated tone to express the disruptive and exacting quality of receiving the GBM diagnosis for *both* Lubbock and herself: "The news is given verbally. We learn something. We are mortal. You might say you know this but you don't" she insists, signaling here a transformational correspondence in Lubbock and her experience. "The news falls neatly between one moment and another," she continues; "it is as if a new physical law has been described for us bespoke. … It is a law of perception. It says, *You will lose everything that catches your eye*" (2).

There is a clear consensus between Cavarero and Coutts' perspectives expressed here: if embodied exposure and perception stipulate selfhood and relationality, then GBM's impact is experienced precisely at the level of witnessing the other's particularly virulent forward thrust toward disintegration. For the primary caregiver, this witnessing assumes an absolute demand for what Coutts elsewhere calls "active attentiveness" ("5x15"): "Under [GBM's] illumination there is no downtime and no off-gaze," Coutts insists. "For its duration, looking can never be idle" (2). Relationality and experience in the context of an aggressive terminal illness also exceed Cavarero's and Carel's conceptual parameters. In Coutts' memoir, what Cavarero calls "a truly altruistic ethics of relation" entails stepping in for the body-under-attack in the context of witnessing the other's embodiment being ravaged by an aggressive illness. At a time of the other's peril, relationality adopts the collective "we" pronoun as a strategy of carrying the other. From organizing a common diet for both herself and Lubbock to help him lose weight before his first craniotomy, to giving up her studio and art because her thinking process had been so radically transformed by the demands of GBM on her family; and from organizing vacations and celebratory outings for her family in an effort to make every remaining moment together both pleasurable and memorable, to assuming the role of sole earner and caregiver to both Lubbock and Ev, Coutts consistently adopts the collective "we" perspective to speak of her days and times with Lubbock's illness. But, in so doing, her and Lubbock's relationality is not reduced to empathy, identification, or confusion, which is what Cavarero fears about rhetorical collectivity. Instead, Coutts' perspective oscillates between the collective "we" and the singular "I," signaling shifts among multiple and dissonant layers of perception. Two among many other moments in her book come to mind.

The first comes early in Lubbock's illness and is a description that Coutts gives of the chronic insomnia that results from the dexamethasone (steroid medication) that Lubbock takes to reduce the swelling in the brain. She notes "We have tried sleeping separately. That didn't work and anyway we want to be together. We can be more inventive than that" (57). The cost of guarding the intimacy of physical proximity through Lubbock's insomnia, for Coutts, is compounded exhaustion. Worrying about GBM's effects on Lubbock and the family unit at large already compromises her physical and mental reserves: "Nights are endurance courses over the distance," Coutts notes. "We endure continuously everything all at the same time." And then, as she restores the singularity of her and Lubbock's individual contexts, she confesses "I am a saint, I tell you, in what is expected of me here. It is a monstrous evil this sainthood. A deformity. Worn like a caul" (59). Another moment in her memoir comes in the final summer of Lubbock's life, soon after his scans show that the chemotherapy regimen accompanying the second craniotomy is not working, and a bout of colitis lands him in the hospital, in isolation, for a six days. When Coutts is allowed to visit him after those six days he appears confused, with a low morale, refusing to leave the hospital in fear of being unable to cope with the conditions at home. "I pretend not to be astonished," Coutts writes. "I edit my voice to keep the surprise out of it but my heart bangs in my chest. What is this? He is changed" (138). And she continues:

One phenomenon irritates me beyond sense. He will not look at me ... does not meet my eye. His voice is dull and without colour. *I am over here*, I keep saying. *Hello. I am here. Look at me!* I wave at him rudely inches from his face. I am belligerent because I am afraid. ... I tell him he has Stockholm syndrome and the hospital is his captor but he scarcely rises to this drollery. ... In the end Tom creeps out of the ward, his face stony, warding me off as a potential foe. But ... as we exit I can feel the man next to me returning, his resurgence following the curve of the roundabout, his body bending softer into the seat as we stream out of the slip road in the direction of home. He winds down the window. *Ah yes*, he says. *Ah yes*.

(139–140)

These two instances, among countless others, capture how Coutts' relational solidarity does not preclude separation, ambivalence, resentment, or even manipulation, if manipulation is the right term for describing Coutts' adherence to Lubbock's earlier expressed desire—"prolong, prolong"—which he comes to overlook as his illness and its cognitive impairment progress. In Coutts' writing Cavarero's ethic is adapted to the context of illness narrative and the patient–caregiver relationship to denote an ethical symbiosis that struggles to retrieve exposure and recognition from the throes of GBM's progression, notwithstanding the affective toll of such effort for the patient and the caregiver. With two-thirds of Coutts' memoir dedicated to the final six months of Tom's illness, the readers of *The Iceberg* get an extensive look at how the enveloping opacity of the illness's final stages directly impacts on the possibilities and limits of Lubbock and Coutts' interdependence and synergy, made most obvious, perhaps, through the progressive collapse of Lubbock's language.

The ultimate conundrum of autothanatography is that you can never be present at your own death to testify to it, Jacques Derrida has said. The same goes for the "obliteration" of consciousness and body from GBM, to repeat Coutt's term for what she was called to witness as Lubbock's primary caregiver. The closest we get to writing that resembles Lubbock's proximity to this obliteration is the final entry in his book, dated October 2010. This entry, Coutts tells us in her introduction to Lubbock's memoir and in her own book, was a piece that was commissioned by *The Observer* and necessitated Coutts and two other friends working as Lubbock's amanuenses for the entire month of October ("in these violent days on the cusp of everything collapsing," says Coutts), to decipher and transcribe what Coutts perceived to be Lubbock's language (178). "At a certain point I became his mouthpiece," she notes, "although without being his brain I was a fraud" (Lubbock, 3).[12] The piece, all 357 words of it, is hauntingly elliptical, its opacity an indication of the annihilation underway. "My true exit may be accompanied by no words at all, all gone," says the narrator of the piece, a fragment of several consciousnesses at work (144). And he proceeds:

The final thing. The illiterate. The dumb.
Speech?
Quiet but still something?
Noises?
Nothing?
My body. My tree.
After that it becomes simply the world.

(144–145)

When we turn to Coutts to witness Lubbock's obliteration, we get a much clearer sense of the effects and impact it produces, once more confirming the verity of Cavarero's analysis for illness writing, namely, that narrative selfhood, by virtue of depending on the other's recognition of one's exposure, depends on the other to tell its story. "Today as he stands mid-morning by the kettle chatting and making tea," begins Coutts' sentence that marks the start of Lubbock's loss of language, "his language trips into rhythmically correct nonsense. It is ludic, quickly recoverable, but it does not sit either with his fits or with his usual slippages and we note the difference in its texture immediately" (90). When a week later Lubbock has a scan to monitor the progression of his GBM they discover that "the tumour is growing again" (91). From that point onward Coutts' memoir starts to track the progress of separation that accompanies the gradual loss of language alongside GBM's growth, a progress whose simultaneous ordinariness and anguish she captures in her description of the present continuous in the context of rapid deterioration: "How many times do I think, *Now we are really in trouble*. ... And this time I mean it more than all the previous times. But there will surely be another time when I will mean it more still and this time will seem ... manageable or benign in retrospect" (122–123).[13] In intervals between seizures, surgeries, chemotherapy sessions, and scans, Coutts monitors Lubbock's unsteady withdrawal even as she remains unsure of how to measure what she witnesses when it is as imperceptible as an absence: "I have empirical evidence but cannot interpret the data," she says. "How to separate companionable silence from withdrawal?" (165). When they try to establish a pattern of communication, Coutts notes how quickly it dissipates, leaving only "the connective tissue of conversation" behind (180). "I taste the idea of separation," Coutts explains, " and the weakening of our orbit around each other and the taste is bitter" (249). As Lubbock worsens he begins to be removed from medical conversations, moving subtly from being talked *to* as a patient to being talked *about* in conversations between doctors and his caregiver. Eventually we find him panicked and grief-stricken as he loses Coutts' and his son's names from his vocabulary weeks before his physical deterioration signals that he must leave his home. The third, penultimate section of Coutts' memoir captures the final two months of Lubbock's life, when his deterioration becomes rapid. As she attends to Lubbock's growing stillness and eventual residency at Trinity Hospice on Clapham Common, Coutts shifts away from the temporal dissonance she has had to negotiate and begins living in a time with "no point of reference, no signs or markers" (275). It is here, in this no-time space, when she can begin to allow for the intimacy that has bound her and Lubbock to come undone. When Lubbock altogether slips from consciousness and language in his final days, Coutts becomes aware that the event she and Lubbock had been anticipating is there for her only and not for both of them. "I have lost the second consciousness that powers mine," she admits; "I am down to one" (287). And she adds "Tom is already elsewhere, gone on his own sometime in the last days" (289). Coutts' own language becomes denser and more poetic than it had been before (it restores its descriptiveness briefly to account for the whereabouts of Ev) and elliptical in its own right. Her memoir concludes at Lubbock's burial site a few pages later: "I scatter earth over you and so does he, fingers splayed back palm flat. You have moved through us and now you are gone, leaving us standing. And so are the living comforted" (294).

Until Further Notice I am Alive and *The Iceberg*, respectively written by an art-critic patient and an artist caregiver, have a compositional affinity with literary artworks in that they invite a reading experience which resists identification and assimilation, even by those of us who have also witnessed the obliteration of a loved one by GBM. Lubbock's parting words referencing the world and those of Coutts referencing the living are provisions for and invitations to a greater inter-relationality, the parting gestures of a dying self and a caregiver bereft. The "world" and the "living" can be read as pertaining to Coutts and their son and their community of friends that attended to the family's needs during Lubbock's illness, but the terms also relate to the readers of Lubbock's and Coutts' memoirs, who have experienced these texts moving through us and upon concluding leaving us standing. Interrelationally entangled in a temporality of shock and crisis themselves, the two memoirs attend to the opacity of Lubbock's illness irrespective of its daunting density and its implications for each of them. What each of them alone and both together are working through is what Peter de Bolla has described as the predicament of duration in affective experience, whereby the singularity of an experiential transformation can only be recognized in its aftermath, not in its immediacy. The unavailability of duration in Lubbock's writing and Coutts' choice to resist its retrospective discernment in her memoir, allow the two texts to explore the transformational experience of illness without retreating to an identity-bound language that establishes a coherent narrative subject or trajectory. That does not prevent them from mattering to the world and to the living, however.

"The particular quality of an encounter with art," de Bolla writes:

> is our coming to understand what we cannot live, what is outside the domain of experience. Yet such encounters feel as if they open a terrain, give onto a clearing in which something like experience seems to happen. But not *to* us, not as part of a continuum of our senses of being, but *through* us, as if the work itself marks us, touches us. ... The materiality of an art response is the virtual sensation of the artwork as a way of knowing. I cannot live that response as an experience, but this does not imply that the experience cannot happen through me.
>
> (35)

Conceived as artworks, Lubbock's and Coutts' memoirs take the temporal elusiveness of the GBM experience, in all its violent, transformative force, and use it to shape the narrative identities of two unstable creatures that go by the generic—collective—designations of "patient" and "caregiver." The opacity that each of their respective writings displays about the experience associated with these identities and their interrelation, captures wordlessly the truth of the shock that is a terminal diagnosis and the obscurity of existence—sense of selfhood—that follows on its heels. "That is a ridiculous question," Lubbock responds to the nurse who asks him to rate his quality of life nearly two months before he dies. "Obviously on a daily basis we go—Oh God, Oh God, Oh God, all the time at all the stuff to be done. But, generally, generally, it is wonderful. We are interested" (207). To read Lubbock's and Coutts' memoirs does not illuminate what is outside the domain of our experience any more than it illuminates the experience of GBM for their authors, though we attend to the writing in the same way Lubbock and Coutts attended to it: we, too, are interested in the "exposure" Cavarero has spoken of, in all its guises. *Until Further Notice I am Alive* and *The Iceberg* mark and touch us by offering themselves as clearings in which we can attend to a process of knowing that is neither tangible nor supplementary, but rather moves through us, leaving us standing, in an other way. In so doing, Lubbock's and Coutts' writing engages the opacity that incurs and sustains some of the most important ethical bonds in the world and among the living, as another mode of knowing and relating to the transformative experience of illness.

Notes

1 The concept of the "Wounded Storyteller" was coined by sociologist Arthur Frank in his eponymous monograph, published in 1995, which conceives of illness memoir authors as "wounded storytellers" who find healing through the recounting of their story through a restitution, chaos, or quest motif, and in the process affirming a social ethic. The concept is readily used in medical humanities writing, even though it has received some criticism.

2 S. Lochlann Jain extensively reflects on the politics of statistics and their effects and notes how "statistics render ... a sort of violence by abstraction" (34).

3 If, as Atul Gawande suggests, the vital questions we all ask when serious sickness strikes are "what is your understanding of the situation and its potential outcomes? what are your fears and what are your hopes? what are the trade-offs you are willing to make and not willing to make? And what is the course of action that best serves this understanding?," then GBM is the kind of disease that often strips one of the time and the ability to process these quality-of-life considerations (256).

4 According to Coutts' introduction to Lubbock's memoir, the final entry in the book dated 10 October was in fact composed with the assistance of Coutts for the purpose of being published in *The Observer*, which had commissioned an article on the progression of Lubbock's illness. The final diary entry that Lubbock wrote unaided was dated 26 August 2010.

5 Nancy Miller, who started a blog project ("web diary") called "My Multifocal Life" after being diagnosed with stage 3b metastatic lung cancer in 2011 (see http://nancykmiller.com/my-multifocal-life/), points out how "Cancer, above all, destroys the

ordinary divisions of time through which we take for granted the capacity—however illusory—of severing past from present, present from future. [L]osing the belief that my present was moving me into some kind of future, made me feel that I no longer had a place from which to write" (430).

6 The use of the term "carnality" here refers to Elizabeth Povinelli's distinction between "corporeality" and "carnality," whereby the former is "a juridical and political maneuver" whereas the latter is "a physical mattering forth ... an independent, unruly vector ... within these biopolitics" (7).

7 In a footnote of her chapter "The shock of the new" Laurie Paul writes "Your own death is the ultimate transformative experience, and as such, you are particularly ill-equipped to approach it rationally" (111).

8 According to Paul "When a person has a new and different kind of experience, a kind of experience that teaches her something she could not have learned without having that kind of experience, she has an epistemic transformation. Her knowledge of what something is like, and thus her subjective point of view, changes. With this new experience she gains new abilities to cognitively entertain certain contents, she learns to understand things in a new way, and she may even gain new information" (10–11).

9 The concept of autothanatography is associated with Jacques Derrida's consideration of Maurice Blanchot's *The Instant of My Death* in *Demeure: Fiction and Testimony*, where according to Linnell Secomb he dubs "autothanatographical" the experience of having "a death within ... awaiting its answering death from without" (41). Tasia M. Hane-Devone has added that "the dialogic nature of autothanatography ... include[s] experiences of others' bodies as well as one's own" (105).

10 In the very next diary entry Lubbock insightfully comments on how "prolongation is ... a familiar narrative form. There is the cliff-hanger serial. There is the shaggy-dog. The soap-opera. The tale is spun out, with an ending wanting to be endlessly deferred." And he concludes "my diagnosis belongs to a low or middle genre. Prolong, prolong. Scheherazade—except that the conclusion is known ahead to be different" (108).

11 "5x15" talks revolve around gatherings in specific locations in London, U.K., where five high-profile speakers spend fifteen minutes talking about their work and life. "5x15" is an initiative of journalist Rosie Boycott, Daisy Leitch, and Eleanor O'Keeffe and started in 2010. Coutts' talk took place in the Tabernacle in 2015.

12 The original request from *The* Observer was for a 5000-word article. The final piece, entitled "When Words Failed Me," was 357 words.

13 With this description Coutts sheds light on one of the most convoluted sub-genre categorizations assigned to illness narratives by Arthur Frank, that of "chaos narratives" (the corresponding sub-category in Jens Brockmeier's taxonomy is given the name "the static model"). For Frank, "chaos" narratives, counterposed to the other two models of "restitution" and "quest" narratives, are stories riddled with anxiety, that emplot the experience of illness as unpredictable and changing, focusing on an ever-shifting present reality whose trajectory is unpredictable at best. In Coutts' writing this "chaos" is an integral, if pragmatic, dimension of witnessing the progression of GBM; it is precisely by guarding the opacity of the experience as chaos that Coutts' illness narrative advances a compelling narrative ethic of reading.

Works Cited

Brockmeier, Jens. "Autobiographical Time." *Narrative Inquiry* 10. 1(2000): 51–73.

Butler, Judith. *Giving an Account of Oneself*. New York: Fordham UP, 2005.

Carel, Havi, Ian James Kidd, and Richard Pettigrew. "The Art of Medicine: Illness as Transformative Experience." *The Lancet* 388(2016): 1152–1153.

Cavarero, Adriana. *Relating Narratives: Storytelling and Selfhood.* Trans. P.A. Kottman. New York: Routledge, 2000.

Coutts, Marion. *The Iceberg.* London: Atlantic Books, 2014.

Coutts, Marion. "Marion Coutts @ 5x15," www.vimeo.com/125609475. Video. 2015.

De Bolla, Peter. "Toward the Materiality of Aesthetic Experience." *Diacritics* 32. 1(2002): 19–37.

De Vleeschouwer, Steven, ed. *Glioblastoma.* Brisbane: Codon Publications, 2017.

Frank, Arthur. *The Wounded Storyteller: Body, Illness, and Ethics.* Chicago, IL: U of Chicago P, 2013.

Gawande, Atul. *Being Mortal: Medicine and What Matters in the End.* New York: Metropolitan Books, 2014.

Hane-Devone, Tasia M. "Auto/thanatography, Subjectivity, and Sociomedical Discourse in David Wojnarowicz's Close to the Knives: A Memoir of Disintegration." *Intertexts* 15. 2(2011): 103–123.

Holland, Eric C. "Glioblastoma Multiforme: The Terminator." *PNAS* 97. 12 (June 2000): 6242–6244.

Jain, Lochlann S. *Malignant: How Cancer Becomes Us.* Berkeley: U of California P, 2013.

Lacroix, Michel et al. "A Multivariate Analysis of 416 Patients With Glioblastoma Multiforme: Prognosis, Extent of Resection, and Survival." *JNS* 112. 2(2010): 190–198.

Lubbock, Tom. *Until Further Notice I am Alive.* London: Granta, 2012.

Miller, Nancy K. "Elegiac Friendship: Notes on Loss." *Feminist Studies* 42. 2(2016): 426–444.

Paul, Laurie Ann. *Transformative Experience.* New York: Oxford UP, 2014.

Povinelli, Elizabeth. *The Empire of Love: Toward a Theory of Intimacy, Genealogy, and Carnality.* Durham: Duke UP, 2006.

Secomb, Linnell. "Autothanatography." *Mortality* 7. 1(2002): 33–46.

Vickers, Neil. "Illness Narratives." *A History of English Autobiography.* New York: Oxford UP, 2016. 388–401.

White, Hayden. "The Value of Narrativity in the Representation of Reality." *Critical Inquiry* 7. 1(1980): 5–27.

Afterword—Representation as a Lens

Teaching and Researching in the Health Humanities

Carl Fisher

Health Humanities is many things. It has been a field without a name at least since classical writers such as Hippocrates started keeping narrative notes on the progression of illness during outbreaks of the plague. The classical conception of *mens sana in corpore sano*, a sound mind in a sound body, designated health. The key was the whole person. By contrast, medicine today is less holistic and often isolates elements of an individual. Medical Humanities began as a medical school subject to encourage humanistic perspectives akin to those of Hippocrates in prospective physicians and then, in the form of Health Humanities, moved to encompass a wider range of people involved in the healthcare setting. As a result of these developments, Health Humanities began to be taught in the undergraduate classroom.

Healthcare occupations are the fastest growing sector of the employment market and will be for the foreseeable future. Doctors, dentists, nurses, therapists, social workers, physician assistants, public health officials, healthcare administrators, and health educators are all in high demand. With the expansion of medical and health education, practices and processes undergo continual development. There are always new sites, situations, and emergent needs. Health Humanities provides historical and cultural contexts for clinical practices and even the implementation of practical skills. Health Humanities emphasizes attention to multidisciplinary viewpoints, including the study of psychological and sociocultural perspectives, and strives to develop skills of observation, analysis, empathy, and self-reflection.

Too often, social skills are not seen as a critical ability, as Dr. Nirmal Joshi notes in a *New York Times* Op-Ed: "The need to train and test physicians in 'interpersonal and communication skills' was formally recognized only relatively recently, in 1999, when the American Board of Medical Specialties made them one of physicians' key competencies" (A17). Since then, the Health Humanities' focus on sociocultural perspectives has had a significant impact on medical education. Not only has the field become recognized both as a scholarly area and as a curricular concentration adjunct in clinical schools, but many colleges and universities now have defined undergraduate programs in the Medical or Health Humanities, whether as a major, a minor, or a concentration. A 2017 study from the Hiram College Center for Literature and Medicine, compiled by Sarah Berry, Erin Lamb, and Therese Jones, shows steady and ongoing growth in these programs. The study documents a range of program names, from the traditional Medical Humanities (more pre-medical school oriented) and Health Humanities (more pre-professional baccalaureate) to "Medicine and Society" (Virginia Tech), "Health and Society" (Beloit College), "Patients, Practitioners, and Cultures of Care" (University of Texas at Austin, listed as being in development for 2019), and "Healing and Humanities" (University of Missouri, Kansas City), just to mention a few examples.

When I first discussed proposing a Medical/Health Humanities program at my university in 2015, an administrator was enthusiastic about the content but dismayed by the program name. He told me that having "Humanities" in the title would be the kiss of death. Despite this myopic view, one of the most vibrant aspects of the field is precisely how it refocuses the purpose of the humanities and the tools of liberal arts training and brings them to bear on the medical/healthcare nexus. It might be a cliché, but the term "healing arts" as a term for medicine is worth exploring because it suggests not just technical mastery but also the compassionate side of treatment. Individuals cannot be reduced to the types of facts, numbers, or data that are recorded in the medical chart; blood pressure, cholesterol levels, and the presumably objective indicators of health status need to be contextualized with the patient's life narrative in order to achieve true meaning. Health Humanities strives to create a sense of a whole being; this holistic perspective also allows a way to understand the experience of others and to develop tools for empathy. Medicine and healthcare are not just healing arts but intimate and personal interactions.

Much of the research in Health Humanities, and the theory behind teaching it, are manifest in specific assumptions, the primary one being that the discipline provides an important adjunct to the technical skills critical for providing care. Nobody doubts that a health professional needs the tools of their trade. Still, social analyses can allow new perspectives, histories have a cumulative effect, philosophy encourages reflection and enriches practice, and representation has impact. Issues of past discrimination, concerns related to implicit and unconscious bias, difficulties in gaining access to adequate healthcare, become narratives told through many disciplinary lenses. Health Humanities tools help to manage expectations, encourage communication in medical settings, provide information, and avoid the strictly clinical.

Being skill-proficient as a provider is essential, but not enough. Here is an analogy that anyone who teaches can understand. You can be a world expert on your subject, but if you are unable to articulate your experience, insight, and passion for the subject to an audience, it is significantly less valuable. For a doctor, making a diagnosis should include empirical inquiry that incorporates the qualitative as well as the quantitative and the ability to communicate this coherently to the person it impacts. If a patient does not understand or if they feel patronized, they might not take their medication, follow up with visits, or address their health concerns. Nirmal Joshi's *New York Times* Op-Ed, cited previously, reports that "one survey found [that] two out of every three patients are discharged from the hospital without even knowing their diagnosis. Another study discovered that in over 60 percent of cases, patients misunderstood directions after a visit to their doctor's office" (A17). Beyond quantification and data analytics, incorporating humanistic perspectives in medical education can lead to a skillset of better communicative strategies and more empathetic responses. Patient satisfaction accrues when a patient is not depersonalized, Joshi notes, which leads to statistically significant better outcomes, often in unexpected areas such as heart attack effects and pneumonia results.

Of course, an important question is how to get these points across and encourage better practices. When I created a "Medicine and Literature" class twenty years ago, the subject was not considered essential to healthcare training. In fact, colleagues made jokes that "Medical Humanities" was an oxymoron. I tentatively offered a class, not knowing if it would even get adequate enrollment. I was surprised when it was the first course to fully enroll in my department the first semester and in all subsequent semesters. Even though students, especially in non-humanities disciplines, might have seen the class mainly as a resume builder, the classroom was vibrant and engaged. I often start my class in "Literature and Medicine" with a poem. After all, what does an undergraduate like more than a poem! The poem could vary—Raymond Carver's "The Autopsy Room," Linda Pastan's "Five Stages of Grief," Rafael Campo's "What the Body Told," Heather McHugh's "What Hell Is," Pablo Neruda's "Larynx"—but given that poetry is a foreign language for many students, it had the benefit of forcing them to attend to something that could not be easily rendered recognizable by Google Translate. A poem cannot (usually) be understood through literal reading or reduced to an obvious formula. A poem is not about plot, although it might have one; it is not about form or structure, per se, although it has a discernible shape. The aspect that makes most students shy away from poetry is that they are sure they are reading it wrong. A good poem, an intense poem, is about messy, complicated, deeply ambiguous aspects of life and, typically, interpreting a poem does not lead to a single "right" answer. Despite macabre themes in these poems—trauma, illness, mortality—or perhaps because of them, students could not look away. There was a level of authenticity to the voices that maintained attention, a reality to which students could relate.

But first, a step back. Like every university instructor who works in a classroom climate framed by trigger warnings, I want to explain a bit more. The poem is not the first thing that the student receives upon attending the class. The exercise in poetic interpretation is set up with an introduction on the first day that outlines class topics and materials and what constitutes the Health Humanities perspective. We discuss how dealing with health and medicine are universal human experiences which span time and cross cultures. We walk through the broader contours of the class syllabus—fiction, interviews, memoirs, cultural studies texts, poems, as well as the supplemental art imagery and film examples—about individual illness, public health concerns, healthcare sites and circumstances, crisis intervention, disability, sexuality, aging, mental health, empathy, and ethics. We discuss how these topics intersect, and how representation can scrutinize the complex relationship between medical practice and human experience. Representations across cultures and in various economic and social contexts are considered crucial to the broader goal of developing ways of building interpretation. The course anticipates sustained discussion of gender roles, social class, and ethnicity, and intends to open a progressive discussion of difference. The essential thesis of the class is that the arts provide a reader/viewer both opportunity for identification but also some distance for judgment in considering essential elements of the human experience.

Thus, there are no surprises about the class themes and topics. Through class discussion and writing assignments, students are encouraged to develop critical thinking skills in relation to medical and healthcare issues, and textual analytical skills through the study of literature and the visual arts, which will help them engage issues they may face as they continue in their academic career as well as in professional occupations. After all of this build up, in what must seem like a letdown, they are given a poem to read before the next class, one of the ones mentioned above, and expected to write a paragraph analyzing it. Despite the weighty themes of the course, and the unexpected nuisance of having to read poetry, rarely does any student drop the class. It probably helps that I include some pop culture, for contrast. A show like *Grey's Anatomy*, as entertaining as it might be, works in the realm of stereotypes in the broadest sense and lacks complexity. Students notice this, either when it is pointed out to them or in reaching their own conclusion. I would not say that they stop indulging in pop culture—that is not the goal of the course—but they can develop tools to consume it with a critical eye.

I switch the course materials on a regular basis, using different stories, novels, and cultural studies, as well as medical journalism—there is always a "new" crisis which filters through a few months of the semester's news cycle—and this highlights the relevance of the readings and connects to the underlying themes of the class. Unlike other classes in my repertoire, all of which I have taught with equal enthusiasm and gusto—about cultural production within traditionally defined literary periods (eighteenth-century studies, Romanticism), broad genres and themes ("Tragedy," "Comic Spirit"), historical literature surveys (world literature, or any national literature)—students seem to find something essential in "Literature and Medicine" that speaks to their common humanity. Students always connect to the texts, whether the work was written about the scourge of medieval plague or the gendered representations of hysteria. Perhaps my perspective is pedagogical hubris. The course might simply fit the right pattern of general education or elective credit. But the level of student preparation and engagement always seems stronger, the class discussions more vibrant, the willingness to debate ideas and deal with ambiguity genuine. The class materials emphasize understanding discourse interference—the conflict between specialized clinical/medical discourse and the broader, highly personalized, deeply politicized, and often melodramatic language of debates regarding healthcare issues. Students connect with this perspective and appreciate the perpetual relevance.

I often focus on how narrative and representation create an empathic space, representing not objectified subjects or patients but often inarticulate people caught in disruptive situations beyond the norms of their daily lives, due to intimidating authority, institutional bureaucracy, unexpected occurrences, or socially inflicted stigmatization—and how authors and artists (and for that matter, many social justice-oriented social scientists) encourage movement toward personal empowerment. We discuss the personally and socially destructive effects of misinformation, miscommunication, and repression on both individuals and communities. We read stories about the behaviors of doctors, often written by doctors, and discuss how important it is for healthcare professionals to deal with their own responses to bereavement and to recognize diversity and enact culturally aware practices. We look at the sociocultural determinants of health and discuss the outcomes on a broad scale and at the individual level. Narratives from around the world are read side-by-side with reports from the World Health Organization to explore the correspondence between what people express and what demographics and geographies demonstrate. Focused topics include public health issues, at-risk and underrepresented communities, nutrition, environmental health, integrated selves, body image, natal practices, end of life care, the many branches of trauma, and healthcare through the lifespan: I actually created another course entitled "Cradle to Crypt" which focuses on this concept exclusively. All these themes and topics are rich in representational examples and provide an opportunity to see medical and health issues from a new perspective.

How did I develop this particular teaching enthusiasm? Not surprisingly, it unfolded along with my scholarship, and in relation to developments in the Health Humanities field. Research has boomed in Health Humanities, archives are devoted to it, and associations have grown around it. The Modern Language Association has multiple discussion groups, and the American Comparative Literature Association runs multiple panels at the annual conference that have Health Humanities cores. Internationally, many scholarly organizations highlight this field. My doctoral area was eighteenth-century studies, and my dissertation was very much about social organization. I researched and wrote about crowds and riots—their definition and their representation—which led me to developing a scholarly interest in graphic images and engravings which depict unflatteringly what Alexander Pope in *Imitations of Horace* (1733) called "the many-headed beast" of the riotous popular body—in other words, the poor, the marginalized, and the voiceless.

While there is not a direct line in my research from crowd scenes to medical representation, graphic satire provided a link. Images of doctors (usually "quacks") and medical treatments (usually detrimental) abound in eighteenth-century graphic satire, and from there my interest in visual culture led to graphic novels and the ways in which these texts flipped the straightforward satiric image (and the narrative implication) of the observed and the observer, the powerless and the powerful, to one that could deal in a complex way with the perspective of the self. Graphic novels about trauma, chronic disease, terminal illness, or bereavement provide historicity, specificity, and individuality. People want to tell their stories and people want to hear those stories; the genre explores the synergy and bridges the space between expressive need and market force.

Graphic narratives with health and illness cores are fascinating to research and equally fascinating to teach. Students read them avidly and attentively, adding interpretations that show an engagement with the medium and an openness to see other points of view. At an age when peer pressure is intense and the "tyranny of the normal" (Leslie Fiedler's term, slightly out of context) is a primary factor in behavior, graphic narrative offers a new way of seeing and feeling outside the self. Graphic narrative may seem an odd way to encourage engagement in medical themes, but the premise that showing, telling, seeing, listening, understanding, and identifying with others develops competencies in professional settings is implicit in Health Humanities perspectives. An entire subfield within Health Humanities has flourished with respect to graphic narratives and has been codified in the *Graphic Medicine Manifesto*, which asserts that the field "arises out of a discomfort with techno-medical progress, working to include those who are not currently represented within its discourse" (Czerwiec et al. 3). Other aspects of the book's argument include that graphic medicine is disruptive to the presumed objectivity of healthcare treatment, and that comics are an outstanding genre for effectively exploring cultural norms and representing taboo subjects.

As graphic novels have found a footing in the market, they have also become an area of scholarly research. Topics I have found particularly engaging for research are those dealing with the representation of socially stigmatized health issues, the self-expression of those figuring out ways to cope with illness or trauma (and the trauma of illness), and the impact of disease on a patient's family and friends. These representations allow an exploration of the ramification of personal beliefs and cultural assumptions about health and illness. Another theme gaining traction is the inner life of doctors, showing how those who enter the medical professions deal with the mechanics of the treatment paradigm, including the physical and psychological effect that it has on them. Often these narratives are written by doctors, and like all self-conscious works, these narratives allow the reader to see from the position of the author/artist/narrator.

Once you start to see how almost everything can be interpreted through a medical lens, the problem becomes not too little material but too much. But that is a good dilemma to face. Texts that embrace the subject, whether they are narrative, visual, or scholarly, participate in cultural conversations, drive medical education, encourage not just technical skills but humanistic traits in medical professionals, through all levels of the hierarchies and the many sites of healthcare. The themes and topics can be sobering, but that they are being addressed is exciting. Change might or might not happen immediately, especially with ingrained perspectives, practices, and habits, but Health Humanities research and teaching creates space to highlight the fundamental humanity at the heart of medicine and healthcare.

Scholars often research cultural phenomena that may not have extensive cultural penetration, but that is why the work needs to be done. A prime example would be eighteenth-century enlightenment projects. How many people actually read the *Encyclopédie*, whether in the time of production or since? But this work has had a lasting influence and continuing intellectual and cultural reverberations (and the value, or the biases, can still be debated). This is how I conceptualize Medical and Health Humanities, as complementary to medical and health education, not antagonistic to it. The field, with all of its permutations, encourages new attitudes and understandings to enhance lives. This type of inquiry recognizes the past and present and provides a vision for the future—a new lens. Researching (and teaching) through the interdisciplinary, intertextual processes of the Health Humanities adds to the toolkit of healthcare to facilitate understanding and promote better outcomes for both patients and practitioners. By including humanistic perspectives into medical and health education, the next generation can see a better way forward.

Works Cited

Berry, Sarah, Erin Gentry Lamb, and Therese Jones. Health Humanities Baccalaureate Programs in the United States. www.hiram.edu/wp-content/uploads/2017/09/HHBP2017.pdf.

Czerwiec, M.K., Ian Williams, Susan Merrill Squier, Michael J. Green, Kimberly Rena Myers, and Scott Thompson Smith. *Graphic Medicine Manifesto*. University Park: Pennsylvania State UP, 2015.

Joshi, Nirmal. "Doctor, Shut Up and Listen." *The New York Times* 5 January 2015: A17.

Index

Page numbers in *italics* indicate Figures.